Getting the Board on Board

What Your Board Needs to Know About Quality and Patient Safety

Third Edition

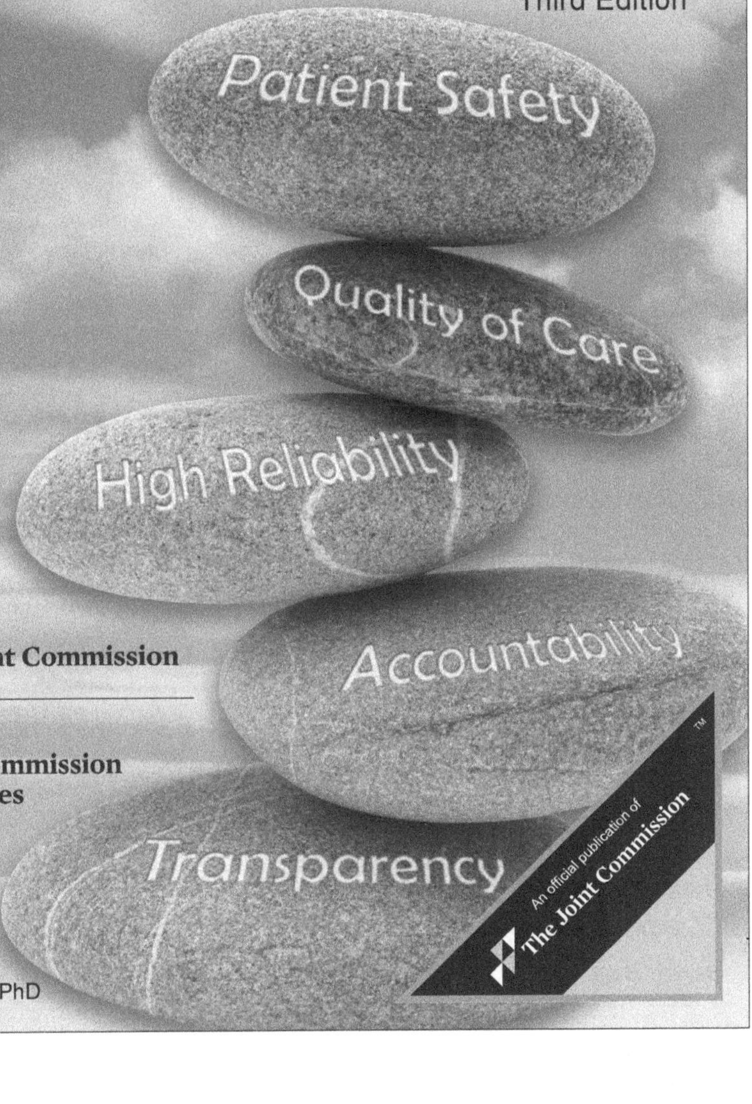

The Joint Commission

Joint Commission Resources

Foreword by
Paul H. Keckley, PhD

An official publication of The Joint Commission™

Senior Editor: Holly Vossel
Content Development Manager: Lisa K. Abel
Project Manager: Lisa M. King
Associate Director, Publications: Helen M. Fry, MA
Associate Director, Production and Meeting Support: Johanna Harris
Executive Director, Publications and Education: Catherine Chopp Hinckley, MA, PhD
Joint Commission/JCR Reviewers: Dima Awad, Ann Scott Blouin, Katie Byrne, Maureen Carr, Jeff Conway, Giovanna De Chiara, Jenna Gillette, Catherine Hinckley, Matthew Icenroad, Carrie Mayer, Jeannell Mansur, Ana McKee, George Mills, Coleen Smith, Sharon Sprenger, Amy Stoefen, Lisa Waldowski, Ron Wyatt, Frank Zibrat

Joint Commission Resources Mission
The mission of Joint Commission Resources (JCR) is to continuously improve the safety and quality of health care in the United States and in the international community through the provision of education, publications, consultation, and evaluation services.

Joint Commission Resources educational programs and publications support, but are separate from, the accreditation activities of The Joint Commission. Attendees at Joint Commission Resources educational programs and purchasers of Joint Commission Resources publications receive no special consideration or treatment in, or confidential information about, the accreditation process.

Joint Commission Resources, Inc. (JCR), a not-for-profit affiliate of The Joint Commission, has been designated by The Joint Commission to publish publications and multimedia products. JCR reproduces and distributes these materials under license from The Joint Commission.

Printed in the USA 5 4 3 2 1

Requests for permission to make copies of any part of this work should be mailed to
Permissions Editor
Department of Publications and Education
Joint Commission Resources
1515 W. 22nd Street, Suite 1300W
Oak Brook, Illinois 60523 USA
permissions@jcrinc.com

ISBN: 978-1-59940-941-2

Library of Congress Control Number: 2011920446

For more information about Joint Commission Resources, please visit http://www.jcrinc.com.

Contents

Foreword

The issues and challenges facing America's hospitals, health systems, postacute providers, and health care professionals are unprecedented. Demand for services across the delivery system is increasing as thousands more per day enroll in Medicare, while disease detection and treatment are becoming more complex. Clinical innovations are changing how and where care is delivered. The 16 million in the health care workforce are being asked to do more with less. Medicare, insurers, employers, and Medicaid are cutting reimbursements. And transparency about costs, safety, outcomes, and patient experiences in every provider sector is feeding a seemingly unquenchable thirst for report cards and performance comparisons.

Complicating matters, implementation of the Affordable Care Act, expansion of risks associated with the False Claims Act, changes to physician compensation under Medicare Access and CHIP Reauthorization Act (MACRA), and a myriad of new laws and regulations heighten risks for all providers.

The combined impact of these factors? Volumes are up. Margins are down. Competition is intensifying. Consolidation is accelerating. And the role and scope of responsibility for directors and trustees of these organizations are dramatically expanding.

For boards, the basics remain: setting an appropriate strategy for the organization, securing capital to fund the execution of the strategy, evaluating affiliations and partnerships, and recruiting and retaining competent management. But perhaps most fundamental is the board's increased role in ensuring that the quality and safety of services provided are at the highest level. And the landscape for both is changing:

- ***Quality of care is no longer assumed.*** It's measured by the organization's adherence to industry best practices and clinical outcomes. Credentialing of providers, team-based care coordination models, interdisciplinary collaboration, clinical pathways, medical management, and outcome measurement are requisites. Boards have responsibility for independently verifying that these efforts are operationalized across the entire organization. Understanding key processes and potential gaps in the provision of necessary services is an increasing focus for leaders and board members who bear ultimate responsibility.

- ***Safety is more than incident capture and review.*** Errors in health care are still prevalent and increasingly exposed to the public. Boards must evaluate their organization's patient and workplace safety programs to determine that they are of unquestionable excellence. Boards bear responsibility for assuring their communities that safety is a constant focus marked by measurement of performance against peers, root cause analysis is completed where safety is breached, and continuous improvement is implemented efficiently and effectively.

The implication for trustees and directors is quite clear: The role is more complicated and time consuming. The buck stops with the board. Meeting attendance is only the beginning. Individual study by directors and trustees along with deeper board education collectively are imperatives. And the focus of these learning experiences must extend to surveillance of issues and trends outside the organization's sector.

The Joint Commission is the nation's most trusted health care partner, serving nearly 21,000 health care organizations and programs in the United States. The Joint Commission brings sophisticated approaches to quality and safety built on a 65-year record of service. Its vigilant attention to valid and reliable measures and process improvement methodologies is the steady hand on which health care boards and leadership depend. Its focus on evidence-based process improvements in safety and quality is the gold standard in health care.

In a time of unparalleled pressures for providers, this book from The Joint Commission and Joint Commission Resources is a board's reliable source for direction and support as it seeks to understand increasing demands on it for quality and safety assurance.

Paul H. Keckley, PhD
2016

Introduction

The US health care industry is in the middle of a fundamental transformation. Recent government-mandated reforms are altering the very way health care organizations provide care to their patients.* Figure I-1, on the next page, represents some of the changes that health care organizations are now facing, or should be prepared to face in the near future. The focus has shifted, the expectations are changing, and so too must health care organizations—and their boards.

Moving Beyond Financial Responsibilities

The Affordable Care Act (ACA) is the major driving force behind the bulk of these changes—many of which impact the financial stability of your organization. The ACA abandons the volume-based model of historical fee-for-service reimbursements, and instead ties payments to the quality of care. In other words, if quality is less, payments are reduced. In addition, the law reduces reimbursements to all health care organizations if they don't prevent harm events and readmissions. This is in direct contrast to the previous system, in which organizations would financially benefit from the additional costs of care related to health care–acquired conditions, such as infections and falls. And whereas historically there was a "disproportionate share" system designed to help cover the costs associated with uncompensated care, these payments are jeopardized as state Medicaid plans struggle with budgets. One analysis suggests these payment changes could lead to a $43 billion reduction in reimbursements between 2018 and 2025.[1]

* The term *health care organization* in this book refers to all types of programs/settings offering physical, medical, and behavioral health care. Different programs/settings refer to those they serve in different ways. In this book, the term *patient* includes residents, clients, and individuals served.

FIGURE I-1: The New Reality of Health Care

This illustration represents some of the challenges that health care organizations now face, or should be prepared to face, in the near future. While some of these initiatives have existed previously, many are new realities.

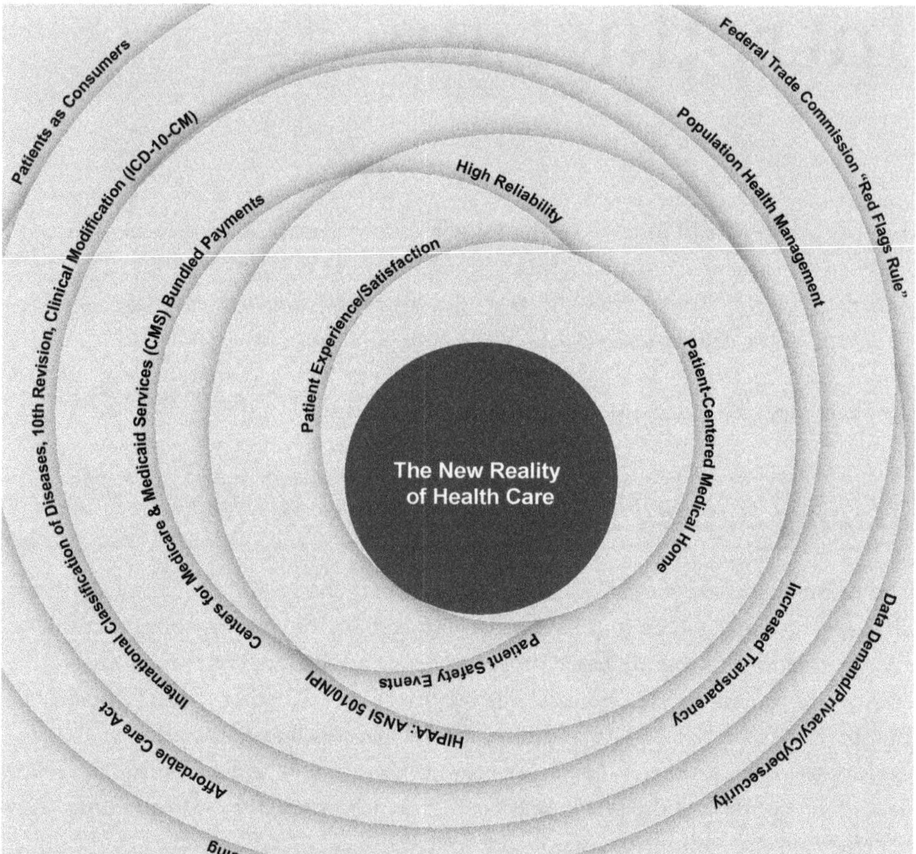

Source: Chassin M, Loeb L. High-reliability health care: Getting there from here. Milbank Q. 2013 Sep;91(3):459–490. Accessed Aug 27, 2016. https://www.ncbi.nlm.nih.gov/pmc/articles/PMC3790522/pdf /milq0091-0459.pdf.

So, beyond the obvious financial impact, what does this all mean for you, a member of a health care organization board?

The Proactive Board

Health care boards are in a prime position to help patient care leaders navigate these tumultuous changes. During these times, you can't have a "business as usual" mentality. You and the other board members must also change. You must be proactive in adjusting your roles, priorities, and structure not only to meet new quality and financial requirements but also to ascertain whether your organization is ready and able to change by meeting quality and safety requirements. In summary, you need to be educated in the newly emerging strategies for success by prioritizing safe, high-quality care.

As a health care organization board member in the new health care reality, you have as much responsibility for the quality and safety within your organization as for its financial surety. Your organization's finances are tied directly to quality; therefore, you must effectively manage quality improvement to effectively manage finances. Government and accrediting bodies require that trustees monitor and responsibly guide quality within their organizations.[2] Ultimately, The Joint Commission, consistent with the Centers for Medicare & Medicaid Services (CMS) Conditions of Participation, views the governing body as responsible for the care and safety of patients. Maintaining current knowledge of this aspect of governance takes time, commitment, and resources.

Purpose of This Book

This book will help you understand the concepts of quality and safety in health care, including why they're such vitally important issues for boards to govern. The discussion will frequently return to the concept of a culture of safety and the underlying need for transparency and accountability that makes safe, high-quality care possible. The purpose of this book is to deepen your understanding and commitment to improving patient safety and quality of care and assist you in carrying out your responsibilities as a board member in relation to quality and safety.

With the rapid changes in health care and consequent changes in board expectations, your resources for addressing such changes need to be fresh and current. Previous editions of this book were best sellers; this new edition includes the best of those editions plus updated information, new case studies, content on high reliability, and more.

Overview of Contents

This book is divided into three chapters, beginning with an overview of quality and safety in health care, moving toward an introduction to The Joint Commission's work in quality and safety, and concluding with specific suggestions about the board's role in relation to quality and safety. Special features appear throughout the book. In addition, the book includes a glossary of relevant terms used throughout the text.

Chapter 1: Overview of Quality and Safety in Health Care Organizations. This chapter begins with a discussion of the board responsibilities for accountability and transparency. This is followed by brief descriptions of the various factors affecting quality and safety, including patient engagement, the ACA, safety culture and communications, and performance improvement. Common areas of concern in quality and safety are addressed next, introducing issues in areas such as fire protection, infection prevention and control, staffing, medication management, emergency management, and hand-off communications. The chapter is rounded off with an introduction to organizations that provide resources and support for quality and safety.

Chapter 2: Introduction to The Joint Commission. This chapter provides an overview of The Joint Commission and how it helps organizations continue to improve quality and safety. The chapter opens with a discussion of the benefits of accreditation and how the Joint Commission standards define the responsibilities of the board. There's a brief outline of the accreditation process, followed by Joint Commission requirements related to performance measurement. Patient safety topics are reviewed, including patient safety events and proactive risk-reduction methods. The chapter concludes with an explanation of the concept of high reliability and how it applies to health care quality improvement.

Chapter 3: The Board's Role in Improving Quality and Safety. This chapter illustrates a series of practical ways boards can actively participate in quality improvement at their organizations. These include putting quality and safety at the top of the board's agenda; creating a quality and safety committee; achieving accountability through transparency, evaluation, and change management; participating in measurement and improvement activities; involving physicians, nurses, and pharmacists as board members; keeping up with regulatory mandates; and engaging in continuous learning.

Special features. Throughout the book, you'll find special features called "Conversation Starters." These features contain questions that board members can ask senior leaders and staff in their organization. Another running feature, "Call to Action," prompts board members to rise to the challenges and lead the charges required for achieving and maintaining quality and safety.

Acknowledgments

The following people provided valuable insights and perspectives in the development of this book by representing the organizations in the case studies featured in Chapter 3:

- Andy Anderson, MD, MBA, Chief Medical Officer – System, and Executive Vice President, Aurora Health Care, Inc., Milwaukee, WI
- Gregg S. Meyer, MD, MSc, Chief Clinical Officer, Partners HealthCare System, Inc., Boston, MA
- M. Michael Shabot, MD, Executive Vice President, Chief Clinical Officer, Memorial Hermann Health System, Houston, TX

We also thank Lea Anne Stoughton for her diligence and patience in updating this edition.

And finally, we would like to extend our gratitude for foreword author, Paul H. Keckley, PhD, for his insight and expertise.

REFERENCES

1. Kaiser Family Foundation. How Are Hospitals Fairing Under the Affordable Care Act? Early Experiences from Ascension Health. Cunningham P, Garfield R, Rudowitz R. Apr 30, 2015. Accessed Aug 23, 2016. http://kff.org/report-section/how-are-hospitals-faring-under-the-affordable-care-act-early-experiences-from-ascension-health-issue-brief/.
2. Health Catalyst. Top 7 Healthcare Trends and Challenges from Our Financial Expert. Brown B. Accessed Aug 23, 2016. https://www.healthcatalyst.com/top-healthcare-trends-challenges/2.

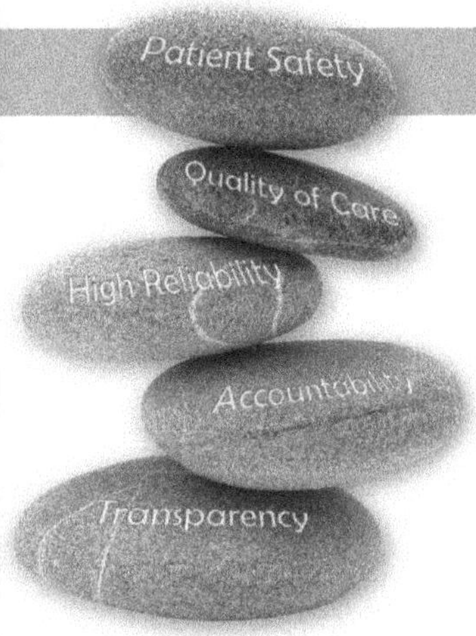

Chapter 1

Overview of Quality and Safety in Health Care Organizations

Every member on your board brings to the table a unique set of skills, knowledge, and experiences. Some board members may be more familiar with medical science, some with finance, others with legislation, and so on. This diversity is valuable. However, health care regulatory and government agencies overseeing your organization put quality and safety of patient care as a top priority. You and the other board members must therefore make understanding quality and safety issues a priority. It's critical to your involvement in improved health for your patients. And it's critical to your responsibilities for high performance on quality and safety measures that link to sound financial health for your organization. The overall success of your organization, in fact, depends on quality and safety, and the organization's board is ultimately accountable for that and for being transparent about it.

This chapter will support your efforts in achieving and maintaining quality and safety by providing an overview of the following:

Board Responsibilities for Quality and Safety
- Accountability via Transparency

Factors Affecting Quality and Safety
- Patient Engagement
- Affordable Care Act
- Safety Culture and Communication
- Performance Improvement

Common Areas of Concern in Quality and Safety
- Infrastructure
- Fire Protection

- Infection Prevention and Control
- Staffing
- Medication Management
- Health Information Technology
- Emergency Management
- Hand-Off Communication

Organizations Helpful to Quality and Safety

- The Joint Commission
- Centers for Medicare & Medicaid Services
- Institute for Healthcare Improvement
- Health and Medicine Division of the National Academies of Sciences, Engineering, and Medicine
- National Patient Safety Foundation
- National Quality Forum
- Agency for Healthcare Research and Quality
- The Leapfrog Group

Board Responsibilities for Quality and Safety

Your organization's leadership, including the board, has serious responsibilities. You must, first and foremost, be accountable to organization stakeholders for quality and safety. These stakeholders include owners and shareholders, staff and other providers, and patients and communities served. You're also accountable to health care regulatory and accrediting bodies. This accountability can be broken down into the following categories[1]:

- ***Mandated accountability:*** Accountability for meeting the requirements of financial, ownership, and regulatory authorities
- ***Voluntary accountability:*** Accountability for meeting the standards of accrediting bodies (such as The Joint Commission)
- ***Community accountability:*** Accountability for meeting the needs of communities and population(s) served

The ability of boards to meet the expectations in each accountability category is becoming more challenging as the health care environment shifts its focus from individual organizational autonomy to systemwide management.[2] But whether your board is responsible to stakeholders in a large or small organization, in a broad or narrow market space, responsibility entails accountability for quality and safety.

Accountability via Transparency

Escalating health care costs as well as mounting alarm over medical errors pose associated accountability challenges: The nation's health care system is under scrutiny, and there's a growing demand for health care organizations to be transparent about performance. Stakeholders want to know if the care being provided is safe, high-quality care—and if not, what's being done to improve it.

Transparency via performance data. Transparency in the form of publicly available performance data has become increasingly mandatory, in part so that patients and purchasers can compare providers and choose those that deliver the most value. Value in health care is a comparison of quality (patient outcomes, safety, and experiences) and cost, often expressed through the following equation: value = quality/cost.

One example of transparency via performance data is reports of adverse events—patient safety events that caused harm to a patient. As of August 2016, 27 states and the District of Columbia have reporting systems requiring health care organizations to report adverse events. Twenty-two of those states report data publicly.[3,4] Many states base their reporting requirements on a list of serious reportable events (SREs) developed by the National Quality Forum (NQF). This list, updated in 2011, contains 29 adverse events that NQF determined are serious, harmful, and largely preventable (*see* page 55).[3,4] The intended goal of NQF's list is to create a standardized national, state-based reporting system.[3,4] This has not yet happened. Incentives for reporting, however, may encourage more voluntary transparency. For example, Medicare (the US government health insurance program) incentivizes transparent reporting through value-based purchasing (VBP) performance programs (*see* pages 21 and 49).

Transparency and community accountability. Clearly, accountability in the form of transparency is now an established expectation for health care organizations. It serves stakeholders for each category of accountability, particularly in community accountability, which is gaining prominence as patients are being encouraged to participate more in their own health on a proactive basis, through smoking cessation programs, healthy nutrition, a physically active lifestyle, and so on. This means that boards must work more with public health, social services, and education agencies not only to determine the health care needs of individuals in the community but also to support preventive health efforts and chronic disease management through patient engagement—and then, of course, to share reports of their performance in these areas.[1] In addition, health care organizations have accountability to the community to be prepared in cases of emergencies and disasters, moving beyond personal health to community health, wellness, and emergency preparedness.

Call to Action
Board Responsibilities for Quality and Safety

Responsibilities for health care organization board members have changed dramatically over the past several decades, becoming increasingly complex and demanding. The Joint Commission standards on leadership, for example, fill an entire chapter in the accreditation manual and define the responsibilities of accredited organizations' board members (*see* Chapter 2 for details on that). You and the other board members who help lead the governance of your health care organizations must take these responsibilities seriously. Board action on needed quality and safety strategies, reliable attendance at board meetings, and rapid resolution of board conflicts that interfere with clear direction to senior leaders are essential for the vital health of your organization.

Factors Affecting Quality and Safety

Patient engagement is just one of many factors you and the rest of the board must learn more about to fulfill your responsibilities for quality and safety. None of these factors is independent of the others, so you need to cultivate an ongoing awareness of them in all their nuanced, integrated forms. A brief introduction to each factor is presented below.

Patient Engagement

The view of patients as passive recipients of care—by both patients and providers—is no longer the prevailing view. Instead, growing numbers of patients (and their families and/or significant others) actively collaborate with and are empowered by their health care providers, as they are willing and able. Consequently, patients are increasingly becoming involved not only in their care but also in their overall health. This becomes even more important with the various settings of care and the transitions that patients experience between levels of care and different care providers. Patients must be engaged and be their own advocates.

Patient engagement impact on quality and safety. Patient engagement is a critical component of patient-centered care, which has been proven to increase quality and safety: Patients who see themselves as respected partners in their care subsequently feel comfortable speaking up when they have questions or concerns. For example, a patient might ask why his or her medication dosage has changed, and by doing so, catch a potentially dangerous error before it results in harm.[5]

Patient engagement initiatives. Patient engagement practices are supported by many organizations through various initiatives and are popular topics in the media. The Joint Commission's Speak Up™ campaign, for example, is intended to inform the public about how patients can help ensure their own safety. The Joint Commission also has standards for providers to welcome and encourage patient engagement and has been involved in books for consumers encouraging patient engagement.* The Questions Are the Answer program and the *20 Tips to Help Prevent Medical Errors* fact sheet, both available from the Agency for Healthcare Research and Quality (AHRQ), are two other well-regarded resources designed to help patients communicate effectively with their physicians. In addition, the Lucian Leape Institute, part of the National Patient Safety Foundation (NPSF), produces free white papers on its website covering a variety of topics—including transparency—so health care consumers can learn what's best for their health care and which organizations can best provide the appropriate care, treatment, and services.

Affordable Care Act

Even before patients began to be more involved in their health care, they were dealing with problems related to paying for that care. In response to those problems, the Patient Protection and Affordable Care Act, also known as the Affordable Care Act (ACA), was signed into law in 2010. This extensive legislation profoundly affects the way the health care industry functions.

More coverage, more care. The primary thrust of the legislation was to expand and reform health insurance coverage, allowing more people access to health care

* Two examples are *The Smart Parent's Guide: Getting Your Kids Through Checkups, Illnesses, and Accidents*, by Jennifer Trachtenberg, MD (2010) and *You, The Smart Patient: An Insider's Handbook for Getting the Best Treatment*, by Michael F. Roizen and Mehmet C. Oz (2006), both books published with The Joint Commission and Joint Commission Resources.

Call to Action
Patient Engagement

As important as it is, patient engagement shouldn't take the place of other quality and safety efforts. It should supplement, not supplant, robust protocols. After all, it's not the patient who's responsible for ensuring safe, high-quality care but rather the organization leadership—including the board. Leadership can and should recognize this component of care by encouraging and promoting patient engagement. One way to do this is to share patient stories at board meetings. Another is to invite patients to participate on improvement committees and projects. You might even consider the appointment of at least one patient member to the board. All of these options are becoming fairly common these days, as are family and patient advisory groups to health care organizations.

than ever before. What does this mean for your organization? It means a higher demand for care and services as patients increasingly take advantage of the opportunities made possible by the ACA's reforms. Sidebar 1-1 on page 19 lists the major reforms. According to the US Department of Health and Human Services (HHS), the ACA has enabled 16.4 million previously uninsured people to gain health coverage, many of those in underserved populations. And uncompensated hospital care costs from uninsured patients were reduced by an estimated $7.4 billion in 2014 alone.[6]

Conversation Starters
Patient Engagement

- *What actions do we take to engage patients in their care?*
- *What are our goals for patient engagement?*
- *How do we measure and benchmark our progress toward those goals?*
- *How do we share our performance in this area with our patients, their families, and staff?*

SIDEBAR 1-1

Major Reforms of the ACA

The reforms contained in the Affordable Care Act (ACA) have been implemented over several years. Listed below are some of the major reforms enacted since the ACA was passed in 2010.

2010

- Ended preexisting condition exclusions for children
- Kept young adults eligible to be covered on their parents' health plans until age 26
- Ended lifetime limits on coverage
- Covered preventive care, such as colonoscopies and mammograms, at no cost to the patient
- Protected the patient's right to choose a doctor from his or her plan's network
- Removed insurance company barriers to emergency services
- Created the Prevention and Public Health Fund to support prevention and public health programs, such as smoking cessation and combating obesity
- Designated funding to expand the number of primary care physicians, nurses, nurse practitioners, and physician assistants, including scholarships and loan repayments for those working in underserved areas
- Increased payments to rural health care providers

2011

- Covered preventive care services, such as annual wellness visits, to seniors on Medicare
- Established a new Centers for Medicare & Medicaid Services Innovation, which tests new ways of delivering care to patients that improve quality of care and reduce the rate of cost increases for Medicare, Medicaid, and the Children's Health Insurance Program (CHIP)
- Improved transitions for Medicare beneficiaries who have been hospitalized, coordinating care between the hospital and community services
- Increased access to services at home and in the community for disabled individuals

2012

- Linked payment to quality outcomes by establishing the Hospital Value-Based Purchasing (VBP) Program in traditional Medicare, which requires hospitals to publicly report performance on measures related to heart attacks, heart failure, pneumonia, surgical care, health care–associated infections, and patients' perception of care

continued on page 20

- Introduced a series of changes to standardize billing and transition to the electronic exchange of health information

2013

- Established a national pilot program that expands authority to "bundle" payments
- Increased Medicaid payments to primary care physicians, requiring states to pay primary care physicians no less than 100% of Medicare payment rates for primary care services
- Opened the national and state-run health insurance marketplaces for enrollment

2014

- Eliminated annual limits on insurance coverage
- Ensured coverage for individuals participating in clinical trials
- Increased access to Medicaid for Americans who earn less than 133% of the poverty level
- Required most individuals to purchase basic health insurance coverage or pay a fee to offset the costs of caring for uninsured Americans

2015

- Modified health care provider payments to reflect the quality of care they provide; those who provide higher value care will receive higher payments than those who provide lower quality care.

Sources: US Department of Health and Human Services. Key Features of the Affordable Care Act by Year. Aug 13, 2015. Accessed Aug 25, 2016. http://www.hhs.gov/healthcare/facts-and-features/key-features-of-aca-by-year/index.html; and US Department of Health and Human Services. ER Access & Doctor Choice. Dec 9, 2014. Accessed Aug 25, 2016. http://www.hhs.gov/healthcare/about-the-law/er-access-and-doctor-choice/index.html.

Reimbursement and quality. In addition to improving access to health care, the ACA aims to improve the *quality* of health care. The law does this by linking government Medicare reimbursements to quality performance metrics, rather than strictly to the volume of services provided. It does this primarily through the following programs:

- ***Hospital Readmissions Reduction Program:*** This program allows Medicare to reduce payments to hospitals with excess readmissions for certain high-cost or high-volume conditions (including heart attack, heart failure, and pneumonia).[7] HHS reports that Medicare all-cause 30-day readmission rates fell to approximately 17.5% in 2013—about 150,000 fewer hospital readmissions among Medicare beneficiaries than in 2011.[8]

- ***Hospital-Acquired Condition (HAC) Reduction Program:*** This program authorizes Medicare to reduce payments to certain hospitals that have a high number of hospital-acquired conditions (HACs) compared to other hospitals.[7] According to HHS, HACs such as pressure ulcers, central line infections, and falls have dropped by 17%, saving an estimated 50,000 lives and $12 billion.[9]
- ***Hospital Value-Based Purchasing (VBP) Program:*** This quality-based payment program affects more than 3,000 hospitals in the United States. Under this program, Medicare adjusts a portion of its payments based on one of the following factors[7]:
  - *Comparative performance:* How well a hospital performs on certain performance measures compared to other hospitals
  - *Improved performance:* How much a hospital improves its performance on certain performance measures compared to a prior baseline period

In addition, the Centers for Medicare & Medicaid (CMS) has launched various "bundled payment" programs. These provide a global payment for all services (including those of physicians and advanced practice providers) for a particular treatment, such as joint replacement.[10]

Tax implications of ACA for nonprofit hospitals. Concern for financial stability is not limited to for-profit hospitals: The ACA has tax implications for nonprofit hospitals. Hospitals categorized as nonprofit must conduct a community health needs assessment at least once every three years to maintain their tax-exempt

Call to Action
Affordable Care Act

The Affordable Care Act (ACA) was a landmark in health care legislation. You and the other board members need to know as much as possible about the impact of the ACA on your organization. Changes to the reimbursement structures, for example, are designed to encourage health care organizations to improve the quality of care they provide. It's imperative that you become aware of these reimbursement incentives and disincentives so that you can help guide your organization. It's particularly important for you to keep in mind as you balance your understanding and oversight of quality and safety with the financial health of your organization.

status. Those that fail to do so face an excise tax. Furthermore, nonprofit hospitals must report to the Internal Revenue Service annually on how they're meeting identified community needs, create a financial assistance policy, and put forth "reasonable" effort to determine whether a patient qualifies for charity care.[11]

Safety Culture and Communication

Patients have always deserved safe, high-quality care—even before becoming more involved in their health care and being better able to pay for that care. To ensure that patients get the care they deserve, an organization must proactively prevent adverse events—and other patient safety events. (*See* Chapter 2 for an explanation of the distinctions among different types of patient safety events.) Of the many proactive approaches to prevent such events, the most fundamental is a commitment from all leadership (including the board and medical staff leaders) to a strong safety culture and effective communication.

Safety culture cycle of trust and transparency. The foundation of any patient safety system is a strong safety culture. Under Joint Commission standards, leaders (including board members) are responsible for establishing and maintaining a safety culture—one in which safety is everyone's top priority. To function, a safety culture needs to be based on mutual trust and transparency. Every participant must be able to report and communicate concerns without fear of reprisal or punishment, even if the concern turns out to be unwarranted. A safety culture thrives when an organization develops a cycle of trust, reporting, and improvement that works hand-in-hand with transparency. As leaders foster trust, staff are encouraged to report events and concerns, which allows the organization to improve. When staff are allowed to see the results of their role in that improvement, it increases their trust, and the cycle continues. (*See* Chapter 2 for information on safety culture components and the relationship of safety culture to high reliability.)

Communication to support a safety culture. Effective communication is certainly necessary to trust and transparency. It's also critical to a safe, functioning environment and safe, high-quality care—the ultimate aim of a safety culture. Poor communication among leaders and staff, among care providers, and among care providers and patients (as well as their families and/or significant others) can result in misunderstood or incomplete orders, wrong or missed doses of medication, and disruption of care when a patient moves to another setting—whether it's to another department, another organization, or home. These potential results of poor communication can in turn lead to patient safety events. Preventing patient safety events is obviously preferable to responding to them if they occur, and overcoming barriers to effective communication is one way to do that.

Language and cultural differences are common barriers to effective communication. Joint Commission standards and common sense require that organizations provide information in a form the patient can understand. This will vary based on factors such as the patient's age, language, disease state, and the ability to understand. But effective communication that breaches barriers is a shared responsibility: Care providers can only work with the information given them. Organizations need to be sure patients know the importance of answering questions honestly, following instructions, and asking questions when necessary. Patients must feel comfortable in sharing potentially sensitive information with care providers and be encouraged to speak up when clarification is needed.

Resources for safety culture and communication. As a board member, you need to lead by example, modeling effective communication behaviors that support a strong safety culture (*see* Chapter 2 for examples of these behaviors). The following are helpful resources to learn more about how to do that:

- ***Sentinel Event Alert, Issue 40:*** "Behaviors That Undermine a Culture of Safety": One of many Sentinel Event Alerts published by The Joint Commission, this one addresses disruptive and intimidating behaviors, examines the root causes of and contributing factors to such behaviors, and suggests actions that can minimize their occurrence. (*See* Chapter 2 for more about these behaviors and about sentinel events.)
- ***Advancing Effective Communication, Cultural Competence, and Patient- and Family-Centered Care:*** A Roadmap for Hospitals: This Joint Commission monograph, available on the Joint Commission website, offers the following:
  - Ways to improve communication with patients and family members at admission, assessment, treatment, transfer, and discharge
  - Guidelines for improving communication with patients and family members when a patient transitions to end-of-life care
  - Description of issues that leadership may face when working to improve communication between hospital staff and patients
  - Practice exercises for each topic that give "how to" information
- ***Oro™ 2.0 High Reliability Organizational Assessment:*** Made available to accredited organizations by the Joint Commission Center for Transforming Healthcare on the Joint Commission extranet, this resource includes a survey tool to assess safety culture. Board members can provide oversight on how

leadership uses this tool to improve the safety culture. The board can review the Oro 2.0 metric and hold leadership accountable for improvements. (*See* Chapter 3 for more about measuring board performance.)

Conversation Starters
Safety Culture and Communication

- *Is disruptive or intimidating behavior tolerated in our organization?*
- *How are such incidents handled when they do occur?*
- *What can board members do to support management in maintaining a safety culture?*
- *What more can the board do to make sure communication is easy and open among patients, staff, management, and leadership?*

Performance Improvement

When a strong safety culture supported by effective communication is functioning well, quality and safety issues will likely come to light. But individual reports of safety issues aren't the primary way they're discovered. Approaches to providing safe, high-quality care have gone through many incarnations in the past few decades. Methods have moved from initial retrospective fault-finding to the introduction of quantifiable measurements in continuous quality improvement and finally to *performance improvement* (PI): The systematic process of detecting and analyzing performance problems, designing and developing interventions to address the problems, implementing the interventions, evaluating the results, and sustaining improvement. The PI process may seem complicated, but that's something of an illusion. The goal is always the same: to make a function or a process better. And the steps are always about the same too. Having different improvement projects going at once in different stages and repeating process steps within those projects is why it may seem confusing.

Performance improvement as a cyclical process. As currently practiced, PI is essentially an approach to examining and improving processes and systems. Most PI methodologies use a cyclical process. Essentially, there are only a few basic steps in that process, as shown in Figure 1-1 on page 26. These are usually repeated for any particular improvement project to make sure improvements are being sustained:

- ***Measure:*** Collect valid, reliable data on a function or process—data about how the function/process is working. Such data typically become part of an internal database.
- ***Assess:*** Analyze collected data and translate information. The information is used to draw conclusions about performance, to identify improvement opportunities, and to set priorities for those improvement opportunities.
- ***Improve:*** Develop, test, and implement certain changes (interventions), either by redesigning an existing process or designing a new one. Define objectives for how the intervention will improve performance.

FMEA and root cause analysis. The Assess step of the PI process often involves benchmarking—comparing performance to tough competitors, industry leaders, or to similar activities in the organization. It also typically includes comprehensive systematic analysis (such as a root cause analysis), and sometimes tools such as failure mode and effects analysis (FMEA). FMEA and root cause analysis differ in critical ways but also share similarities.

- ***Differences:*** The fundamental difference in the two tools is timing. Root cause analysis is a retrospective approach, whereas FMEA is a proactive approach designed to keep unwanted events from occurring in the first place. In other words, root cause analysis asks "Why?" after an event has occurred to identify the root causes of the event; FMEA asks "What if?" to explore what could happen if a failure occurred at a particular step in a process.
- ***Similarities:*** FMEA and root cause analysis have the following characteristics in common: They're both nonstatistical methods of analysis. The goal of both is to reduce the possibility of future patient harm. They both involve identifying conditions that lead to harm. They're both team activities.

Note that The Joint Commission has PI standards that address the PI process. The Joint Commission doesn't mandate which type of methodology a health care organization uses, but they do need to use some PI methodology consistently. And because health care organizations must do PI, the board must embrace it. (*See* Chapter 2 for more about Joint Commission requirements for PI and Chapter 3 for more about the board's role in the PI process.)

FIGURE 1-1: The Performance Improvement (PI) Process

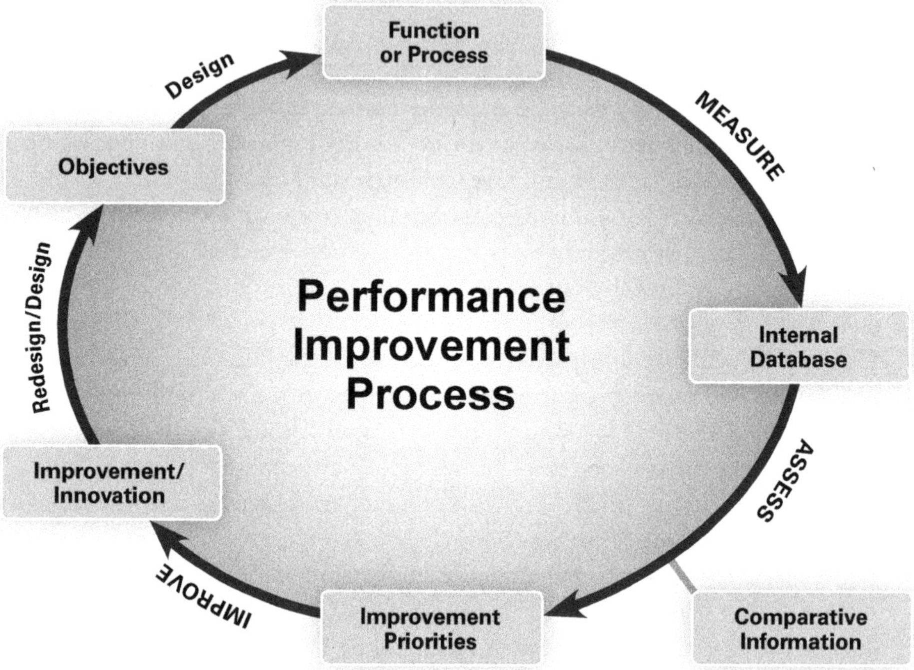

Performance measurement as part of the process. Performance measurement, also a Joint Commission requirement, is clearly a major component of PI. More than just pulling numbers together, performance measurement is a systematic collection and analysis of data over time. It includes the following:

- Choosing valid, reliable measures
- Setting performance goals
- Planning and implementing data collection activities
- Evaluating and comparing data
- Organizing and presenting data in useful ways

Performance measurement reports to the board. As board members, you'll review reports about quality and safety issues, such as falls, restraint use, pressure ulcers, readmissions, and surgical site infections—reports based on performance measurement. These reports should be used by the board as a basis for decision making and prioritization, so the reports must be frequent and comprehensive enough to keep you adequately informed. And it's imperative that the reports be based on reliable, accurate data. (*See* Chapter 2 for more about performance measurement in relation to the Joint Commission accreditation process.)

Performance improvement process models. There are many ways to carry out the PI process. Among the most common models used by PI professionals are the PDSA (Plan-Do-Study-Act) or PDCA (Plan-Do-Check-Act), the Toyota Production System, and Six Sigma's DMAIC (Define, Measure, Analyze, Improve, Control). In addition to these, The Joint Commission has incorporated other tools. Collectively known as Robust Process Improvement® (RPI®), these include evidence-based PI tools from Lean Thinking, Six Sigma, and change management. Health care organizations have increasingly invested in PI training over the past decade. The Joint Commission encourages organizations to do so. (*See* Chapter 2 for more about RPI.)

Call to Action
Performance Improvement

Traditionally, board members may have viewed their responsibilities primarily as strategy and operational guidance regarding the financial health of an organization. However, in a contemporary health care organization that view dramatically underestimates your fiduciary role in quality and safety. One critical component of fiduciary responsibility is learning what, where, how, when, and by whom quality and safety indicators will be measured as well as how performance reports are shared with the board. Reimbursements, remember, are now tied to safety and quality. You're also responsible for reading and responding to the reports, helping to prioritize performance projects, and supporting PI efforts in your organization.

Common Areas of Concern in Quality and Safety

Identifying an area for improvement is a key part of the PI process. This is typically done through an examination of data and/or proactive risk assessment. (*See* Chapter 2 for more about risk assessment.) Safety risks may arise from the performance of tasks, from the structure of the physical environment, or from situations beyond the organization's control (such as weather). And although every health care organization is different, and will have different areas of concern in quality and safety, there are those that are common to most, if not all, organizations. For example, fire protection is a common area of concern for hospitals, nursing homes, and ambulatory surgery centers, while infrastructure, staffing shortages, medication management, infection control, and emergency management can be problematic for all settings along the continuum of care. Consequently, issues related to common areas of concern are frequent topics of PI activities, which the board needs to review. The following sections describe these issues at a high level.

Infrastructure

The aging infrastructure of health care buildings can put everyone in those buildings at risk of an adverse event—and can hamper efforts to improve quality and safety. Many building materials degrade with use and exposure to elements over the years. Aging equipment malfunctions or fails. And both the structures and the equipment often become inefficient and/or inadequate for current needs—including the need to meet updated safety codes. The term *latent conditions* has been used to refer to things built into the physical environment itself through poor design decisions. These can lead to situations creating opportunities for adverse events.

Ongoing research in facility design has led to advances that better support quality and safety. For example, with a new understanding of the causal relationship between reducing patient stress and positive outcomes, facilities are incorporating features to lessen stress, such as appropriate access to positive distractions (particularly nature), noise reduction, and natural light.

Similarly, the importance of building features and equipment to infection control has had a huge impact on facility design. One important component is the number, placement, and design of hand-washing sinks and alcohol-based hand rub dispensers. The move to single-bed rooms has been shown to reduce the risk of spreading infection among patients.[12] Another factor in infection control is achieving and sustaining air and water quality through well-functioning, well-maintained utility systems.

Call to Action
Infrastructure

Organizations have an opportunity during the design phase of construction and renovation projects to anticipate, address, and manage safety risks in new construction or renovation of a health care facility. Boards need to consider how facility design can support or hinder quality and safety when reviewing proposals for renovation or construction projects. Your role in the process is to carefully consider how to balance the benefits of the design against the project costs to ensure that financial and other resources are allocated in ways that will have the greatest practical impact on quality and safety.

Fire Protection

As noted, aging infrastructure poses risks that include the inability to meet safety codes. Some of the most stringent and complex safety codes are those related to fire protection. The serious ramifications of fire are intensified in health care facilities because of the number of people in those facilities who are unable to move independently. The requirements to achieve and maintain a fire-safe environment are therefore particularly challenging for health care organizations to comply with and are a frequent area of concern.

Fire safety vs. life safety. To better understand fire protection requirements from The Joint Commission and other authorities, it's helpful to understand the difference between the terms *fire safety* and *life safety*. In the Joint Commission standards, both terms relate to fire protection and address the minimum requirements for facility systems to offer fire protection; the differences are how that protection is provided:

- ***Fire safety:*** This term relates to fire protection that's dependent on human intervention, such as the use of fire drills and fire safety equipment (fire extinguishers, alarm pull stations) and maintenance of alarm and sprinkler systems. The standards for fire safety are in the "Environment of Care" (EC) chapter of the accreditation manual, which applies to all accreditation programs/settings; they address the way people respond to and intervene in a fire situation.

- ***Life safety:*** This term relates to fire protection dependent on intervention via building features—alarm and sprinkler systems, building construction and design (including location of exits), means of egress (essentially, a clear way to get out of a building from any point in the building), and fire protection hardware. The standards for life safety are in the "Life Safety" (LS) chapter of the accreditation manual, which applies to most accreditation programs/settings; they address how the building structure and its components work in a fire situation. The standards are based on and frequently refer to the National Fire Protection Agency (NFPA) set of codes known as the *Life Safety Code®*.*

Compliance challenges in life safety. Meeting LS standards is a significant challenge for many organizations. Among the more common areas of compliance deficiency are corridor clutter, unsafe projections into the corridor, locked doors in egress areas, electrical overload and power strip use, and smoking and e-cigarettes. Compounding the problem is the difficulty of maintaining safety during special circumstances, such as construction, renovation, or demolition; the reorganization of how the space is used; an incident of accidental damage; or an emergency situation. Even the smallest change can affect life safety. For example, a painting project might involve ladders, buckets, and other supplies cluttering corridors, and possibly turning off or removing exit signs—conditions that would affect the ability of people to exit quickly and safely if a fire starts.

Interim life safety measures. In cases where the exact provisions of the *Life Safety Code* can't be met, your organization must still ensure that safety is maintained. This is done through interim life safety measures (ILSMs). ILSMs must be used whenever a *Life Safety Code* deficiency can't be immediately corrected. The specific activities will vary depending on the situation. Examples of common ILSMs include the following:

- Inspecting exits in the affected areas on a daily basis
- Using temporary construction partitions that are smoke-tight, or made of materials that won't contribute to the spread of a fire
- Conducting additional fire drills
- Providing temporary but equivalent fire alarm and detection systems
- Providing additional firefighting equipment

There are many other ILSM activities that may be used; not all will be applicable to all situations. Your organization should have a written ILSM policy that's adaptable and broad enough to apply to any type of deficiency.

A life safety tool. The Joint Commission provides a special tool to help health care organizations such as hospitals and nursing care centers with the *Life Safety Code*: the Statement of Conditions™ (SOC). The SOC is accessible online to accredited organizations, and walks you through identifying your organization's life safety risks and deficiencies, planning how to address them, and making sure the plan is carried out effectively and in a timely fashion.

Infection Prevention and Control

As noted above, appropriate buildings and equipment are as critical for infection prevention and control as they are for fire protection. In addition to hand hygiene facilities and single rooms, infrastructure measures to prevent and control infection may include decontamination facilities, properly ventilated isolation rooms, and provision of a central department for reprocessing (cleaning, disinfection, and sterilization) of medical equipment, devices, and supplies. Building features need to be sufficient for handling an influx of patients with infectious diseases, such as recent outbreaks of H1N1 influenza, Ebola virus, Zika virus, measles, whooping cough, and various foodborne illnesses that have been widely publicized in the United States and elsewhere. And of course, proper facilities and equipment are necessary to prevent and control infections from multidrug-resistant organisms (MDROs) such as *Clostridium difficile* and methicillin-resistant *Staphylococcus aureus* (MRSA).

Health care–associated infections. MDROs are often the cause of health care–associated infections (HAIs), which remain at the top of organizations' patient safety concerns. According to the most recent estimates from the Centers for Disease Control and Prevention (CDC), there are 722,000 HAIs every year, resulting in about 75,000 deaths.[13] Many types of HAIs can result from ineffective infection control practices in organizations. Some of the most common HAIs are as follows:

- Surgical site infection (SSI)
- Catheter-associated urinary tract infection (CAUTI)
- Central line–associated bloodstream infection (CLABSI)
- Ventilator-associated pneumonia (VAP)
- Diseases associated with environmental pathogens, such as *Legionella* and *Aspergillus*

* *Life Safety Code*® is a registered trademark of the National Fire Protection Association, Quincy, MA.

Various factors can affect HAI rates, including the following:

- Cleaning and disinfection of medical equipment
- Environmental safety
- Observance of standard- and transmission-based precautions
- Annual influenza vaccinations for health care staff
- Hand hygiene practices
- Antibiotic stewardship

Help for hand hygiene. Hand hygiene is the simplest and most effective way to prevent infection. Yet, consistent adherence to hand hygiene protocols isn't so simple; it poses a struggle for many organizations. In an effort to increase hand hygiene compliance rates, the Joint Commission Center for Transforming Healthcare and eight of the country's leading health care organizations developed a Targeted Solutions Tool® (TST®) for hand hygiene. The TST examines the specific reasons health care staff fail to comply with hand hygiene practices, and then offers potential solutions to those barriers that have been successful at other organizations. The hand hygiene TST can be accessed online at www.centerfortransforminghealthcare.org/tst_hh.aspx.

Influenza vaccination for health care workers. Hand hygiene isn't the only area in which staff compliance plays a central role in infection control. Influenza vaccination for health care workers is a subject of much discussion recently. The CDC reports that influenza causes millions of illnesses, hundreds of thousands of hospitalizations, and thousands of deaths each year. Despite CDC recommendations that all health care workers get vaccinated against influenza every year, only an average of about 64% do.[14] The Joint Commission also strongly encourages influenza vaccination for health care workers. Its accreditation standards require organizations to have an influenza vaccination program, educate staff and licensed independent practitioners about the influenza vaccine, and provide influenza vaccination at accessible times and locations. The goal is to maximize the influenza vaccination rates at organizations.

Special populations at risk for infection. Getting health care workers to comply with infection control practices becomes particularly important when caring for patients who are already frail and/or have weakened immune systems. These individuals might include the following:

- Infants
- Elderly individuals

- Patients with compromised immune systems due to disease, such as AIDS or leukemia
- Patients whose treatment compromises their immune systems, such as those undergoing chemotherapy
- Patients in intensive care units (ICUs)
- Patients who have been rendered susceptible to infection by inappropriate use of antibiotics

Every health care organization will encounter some or all of these patient populations. Therefore, a well-integrated plan to prevent and control infections of all types for all relevant populations is fundamental for every organization.

Infection prevention and control plan. An effective infection prevention and control plan involves many activities, including surveillance (identifying potential and actual risks of infection) and reporting of adverse events and PI initiatives. Boards may wish to request data on use of certain types of medical devices that commonly contribute to infection control risks (such as ventilators, central lines, and catheters). Using data like this and other forms of risk assessments, your organization can create a customized plan. Factors such as the type and scope of services provided, the patient population, and the surrounding community all play a part in developing that particular plan. In other words, there's no one plan that's appropriate for every health care organization.

And, although your organization may have an infection prevention and control leader, department, or committee, there's no one person, department, or committee solely responsible for infection prevention and control; everyone in the organization must share that responsibility and participate in infection prevention and control activities. When designing an infection prevention and control plan, therefore, representatives from each area/department should be included and asked for input. This is yet another situation in which the promotion of a culture of safety is essential, because staff must be trained and then encouraged to actively look for and report infection prevention and control issues.

Staffing

Trained staff with the appropriate qualifications and skills are vital to quality and safety in all areas of your organization. A well-staffed facility, with experienced, competent staff, is more likely to have better clinical outcomes, including lower mortality rates, shorter lengths of stay, and reduced costs of care.

Some organizations, however, particularly in rural and underserved communities, are finding it difficult to supply the professional staff their patients require—and the situation isn't going away. The Bureau of Labor Statistics' Employment Projections anticipates the demand for registered nurses to grow by 19% by 2022, with the anticipated number of job openings over one million.[15] Current shortages aren't limited to any particular type of organization or position. Nursing care centers, home health agencies, and ambulatory and behavioral health care facilities are all struggling with staff shortages—from aides to assistants, pharmacists to technicians, and other staff.

Inadequate staffing can create serious problems. For one thing, it puts an increased burden on caregivers, often subjecting them to longer hours, heavier patient load, more paperwork, exhaustion, reduced personal health status, and more stress. Risk to patient safety is also significant when existing staff are spread too thin.

Insufficient nursing staff. When nursing staff are insufficiently available to provide safe, high-quality care, they must make decisions about what care can and cannot be completed. The research on this "missed nursing care" when understaffed is very clear and consistent. For example, patients who aren't ambulated have been shown to be at greater risk of falls, new onset of delirium, pneumonia, pressure ulcers, increased pain and discomfort, and other negative outcomes.[16] Similarly, missing mouth care leads to a patient being reluctant to eat, which in turn increases risk of oral ulcers and/or pneumonia.[16] Other key nursing care components, such as emotional support, patient education, and discharge planning, also suffer or are missed when staffing numbers are inadequate.[16]

In contrast, although there's no federal mandatory nurse/patient ratio, studies have shown that a higher number of registered nurses is associated with improved survival rates among patients in intensive care units.[17] Increased numbers of registered nurses has also been linked to reduced readmissions of cardiac[18] and pneumonia[19] patients.

Insufficient pharmacists. Evidence indicates that, like nurse/patient ratios, effective pharmacist/patient ratios result in positive outcomes. These include increased medication safety, decreased medication errors, and reduced cost.[20] In addition, pharmacist review of high-risk patients' medication treatments is linked to a reduction in medication-related adverse events.[20] This type of review process is inherently patient-specific, and therefore its effectiveness is limited by the number of available clinical pharmacists who have the appropriate skills and training.[20]

Indeed, as the pharmacist has evolved from primarily dispensing medication to taking an active role in managing and optimizing patients' medication therapies, the importance of sufficient pharmacist staffing has grown.

Staff competence and empowerment. Staff/patient ratios, of course, are not the only factors to consider when assessing staffing needs: "More staff" alone is not enough. The qualifications and competency of all staff must be clearly defined and assessed initially and regularly thereafter. It's essential to ensure that staff members have the skills relevant to their job tasks and that they use those skills safely and efficiently. In addition, staff must be assigned and managed in a way that supports a positive, effective work environment, which benefits everyone.[21]

Productivity and job satisfaction increase, for example, when people have a sense of ownership and empowerment in their jobs. Involving frontline staff in evaluating and simplifying processes to help prevent errors promotes this sense of empowerment. It's also practical because the people who know a process best are those who use it every day. Empowerment is yet another example of the benefits of a strong safety culture. And it's a huge factor in retaining staff.

Retaining staff. Recruiting new staff with the appropriate competencies is a challenging process, but the need to retain current staff is a challenge that's often overlooked. From a financial perspective, staff turnover is expensive. For example, one survey estimates the average cost of turnover for a bedside registered nurse ranged from $37,700 to $58,400.[22] When you consider that the turnover rate for bedside registered nurses is 17.2%,[22] it's clear that staff retention makes fiscal sense. More importantly, though, retention of experienced staff leads to higher-quality care and greater safety. The relationship of cost and care is an ever-present one and is reflected in satisfaction scores as well.

Impact of staffing on satisfaction scores. Missed nursing care, as described above, not only results in patients going home or to the next care setting insufficiently prepared but also results in poor patient and family satisfaction.[16] Moreover, nursing staff feel frustrated, knowing that their patients missed key nursing care due to inadequate resources. This results in decreased nursing staff satisfaction and eventually retention problems. Patients and families in turn are affected by this staff frustration, which leads to further lowered patient satisfaction.

Lower staff satisfaction ratings and lower Hospital Consumer Assessment of Healthcare Providers and Systems (HCAHPS) scores have been clearly correlated.[23]

Furthermore, like quality and safety, HCAHPS scores and other measures of patient satisfaction are increasingly tied to reimbursement. Therefore, it's essential that you and the rest of the board evaluate your organization's staffing as a critical component of quality and safety.

Resources for staffing issues. Board members who want to improve their organization's nurse staffing issues can seek out resources such as the following:

- ***Health Care at the Crossroads:*** Strategies for Addressing the Evolving Nursing Crisis: This Joint Commission white paper recommends strategies for creating a culture of retention, enhancing the educational infrastructure for nurses, and incentivizing investment in nursing. It's available on the Joint Commission website: www.jointcommission.org/assets/1/18/health_care_at_the_crossroads.pdf.
- ***The Future of Nursing:*** Leading Change, Advancing Health: This report, published by the Health and Medicine Division (HMD) of the National Academies of Sciences, Engineering, and Medicine (the Academies), makes recommendations regarding overcoming barriers, improving education, and expanding the scope of practice for the future of nursing. It's available on the Academies website: http://nationalacademies.org/hmd/reports/2010/the-future-of-nursing-leading-change-advancing-health.aspx.

Call to Action
Staffing

To meet the patient care demands of your health care organization, you and the other board members have a fiduciary responsibility to understand the adequacy of staffing—both in number and competencies. Asking questions and routinely receiving information about the number, location, and type of vacancies are critical to board effectiveness in this key aspect of human resources. If you want to attract and retain high-quality staff, however, you have to go beyond providing sufficient staff. You need to maintain a work environment that's safe, effective, and efficient. You need to create opportunities for advancement and growth, including those provided by mentoring. You need to ensure competitive compensation and benefits. And you need to foster a strong organizational culture based on common vision and mission.

Conversation Starters
Staffing

- *What positions and how many positions are open?*
- *How long have the positions been vacant, and what recruitment efforts have been made?*
- *What are the turnover statistics?*
- *What do our employee opinion and staff satisfaction surveys tell us?*
- *What are our patient satisfaction scores?*
- *What action plans do we have to address weaknesses in staffing?*
- *What are our plans to increase the likelihood of effective recruitment and retention strategies?*

Medication Management

Medication errors top nearly every health care setting's list of problems, so sufficient numbers of well-trained, competent staff—particularly nurses and pharmacists—are vital to help reduce these events, which are all too common in medication management. The process of medication management encompasses selecting, procuring, storing, prescribing/ordering, preparing, dispensing, administering, disposing, and monitoring medications.

Problems are possible at any point in the process, from incomplete or illegible orders to inaccurate labeling to incorrect dosage. Factors that create problems in medication safety include the following:

- Lack of adequate training and education
- Poorly designed medication management systems
- Medication shortages and subsequent substitutions
- Increased potential for harm with high-risk processes and high-alert medications
- Lack of a robust medication error system to provide actionable intelligence
- Failure to conduct proactive medication risk assessments

Communication in medication management. Good communication is one key to overcoming many challenges posed by problems in medication management. Whether you call them problems or challenges or risks, they'll vary depending on each organization's particular situation. For example, if a hospital doesn't have a 24-hour pharmacy, it will need to contract pharmacy services during off-hours, and communication with that outside company adds risk. If a nursing care center receives many medication orders over the phone, the potential for misinterpretation adds risk. If a home care agency hires someone with language skills that don't match the needs of the patient, communication about medication adds risk. That communication should involve the patient and all care providers along the continuum of care. Yet many medication errors are, at their root, system or practice-model related. These problems include lack of integration or interoperability, technology issues, and incorrect medication orders transcribed or dispensed. The Institute for Safe Medication Practices (ISMP) publishes medication errors reports that highlight these and other challenges at www.ismp.org.

Reporting errors in medication management. Reporting errors is part of the effective communication that's part of a safety culture, as described earlier in this chapter. Your organization must analyze its medication management system to ensure that all patient safety events are actually being captured and reported appropriately—including "close calls"—patient safety events that did not reach the patient. If the reporting system isn't performing well, it can lead to a false sense of security about safety. Having few error reports doesn't necessarily mean that safety is good—it might mean that the reporting system is bad.

Boards might consider requesting reports on serious medication errors as part of their safety-related activities. Those reports are only effective when they're received and addressed through a zero preventable harm or high reliability approach. A highly reliable organization embraces error reports because each one is an opportunity to make adjustments and improve safety. The more "close calls" that an organization captures, for example, the better chance it has to make changes before a patient gets hurt. (*See* Chapter 2 for more about high reliability.)

Root cause analysis of medication errors. If a medication error occurs, the organization should do a root cause analysis. This information is used to inform and direct the organization's PI efforts. The Joint Commission publishes data from its Sentinel Event Database each year that can help an organization better understand potential contributing factors for the errors its reporting program may unearth. (*See* Chapter 2 for more about sentinel events.) An analysis of medication error events reviewed by The Joint Commission revealed the following root causes, in order of frequency, although the majority of medication errors had multiple root causes[24]:

- Medication use (for example, wrong medication, wrong dose)
- Communication

- Human factors
- Leadership
- Assessment
- Information management
- Physical environment
- Health information technology (HIT)–related issues
- Care planning
- Continuum of care

Types of medication management technology. Technology can also help reconcile and otherwise manage medication and help to prevent medication errors. Many technologies interface with medication processes, and it's important to understand how those technologies can affect quality and safety. Designed and used properly, those technologies can support quality and safety efforts. Examples of technological components of medication management include the following:

- Computerized provider order entry (CPOE)
- Clinical decision support tools
- Bar-coded medication administration (BCMA)
- Automated dispensing cabinets (ADCs)
- Medication alarm or alert systems
- Electronic health or medical records (EHRs or EMRs)
- Smart IV pumps
- IV robots
- Medication carousels
- Medication robots
- Medication management and compliance software

Risks with medication management technology. Using medication management technology can help improve communication, allow easier access to key information, provide alerts to possible errors, and other benefits. However, some medication technologies have particular risks that health care organizations should carefully manage. For example, ADCs[25] and CPOEs[26] will alert the user of a potential error. The user can override or dismiss the alert if necessary. The problem is that the sheer number of alerts can overwhelm the user and lead to alert (alarm) fatigue. Thus, critical alerts are dismissed along with the rest. And BCMAs pose other risks. When used properly, they help ensure that the right patient is receiving the right medication. But in the fast-paced health care environment, staff may administer medications before scanning, or miss scanning entirely.[27] These workarounds increase the risk of a medication error.

Health Information Technology

Factors related to health information technology (HIT) are among the top contributors to medication error sentinel events, according to Joint Commission analysis.[24] And medication management isn't the only area affected. In 2008 The Joint Commission issued *Sentinel Event Alert* 42: "Safely Implementing Health Information and Converging Technologies." This publication discusses common safety concerns related to technology, including selecting products to meet organizational needs, planning the impact of new technology on existing care processes or workflow, and maintaining data continuity when new technology is introduced. This publication is available online: www.jointcommission.org/assets/1/18/SEA_42.pdf.

More recently, in 2015, The Joint Commission issued *Sentinel Event Alert* 54: "Safe Use of Health Information Technology." This publication continues the earlier Alert's broad look at the risks involved with HIT. It discusses the types of technology-related errors organizations should address, such as human-machine interface, workflow and communication, and clinical content. It also suggests actions that organizations might take to mitigate these risks, which center on safety culture, process improvement, and leadership. (*See* Chapter 2 for more about these topics.) This publication can be accessed online too: www.jointcommission.org/assets/1/18/SEA_54.pdf.

HIT and "converging technologies." The interrelationship between HIT and medical devices—HIT and "converging technologies"—is of increasing concern in health care organizations. HIT is found almost everywhere: medical devices, EHRs, medical billing, scheduling, laboratory test reporting, diagnostic imaging, and so on. And the information generated by HIT is increasingly interconnected to provide efficient, seamless care across the health care continuum, creating "converging technologies."

Sociotechnical dimensions that affect HIT. Unintended patient safety events related to this relationship typically arise from the design of the human-machine interfaces or processes and workflows associated with the technology. The overall safety and effectiveness of technology in health care ultimately depends on its human users, ideally working in close concert with properly designed and installed electronic systems. *Sentinel Event Alert* 54 identifies eight sociotechnical dimensions that affect HIT. They are listed here in order of their frequency[28]:

1. Human-computer interface (ergonomics and usability issues resulting in data-related errors, such as selecting the wrong option from a drop-down menu)

2. Workflow and communication (issues related to HIT support of communication and teamwork, such as the integration of a system into the process of care)
3. Clinical content (design or data issues relating to clinical content or decision support, such as nurses and physicians not having access to the same parts of the medical record)
4. Internal organizational policies, procedures, and culture
5. People (such issues as lack of training or failure to follow established processes)
6. Hardware and software
7. External factors (such as those originating from the vendor)
8. System measurement and monitoring

Call to Action
Health Information Technology

Organization leaders, such as board members like yourself, are responsible for creating a strong safety culture, which includes ensuring HIT safety. Because HIT involves every functional area of a health care organization, and requires the transfer of data among providers in different departments, you must also provide oversight. Working with other leaders on multidisciplinary teams across your organization, you can gather relevant information that informs decisions on HIT planning, implementation, and evaluation.

Emergency Management

Another factor affecting HIT—and other systems in a health care organization—is the ever-present threat of an emergency. Whether natural or manufactured, emergencies can interrupt an organization's access, utility functions, and ability to provide care. Emergencies can also create a patient surge, which can be complicated by the emergency itself. For example, a severe storm may knock out power, compromise water supplies, block roads, and injure many people.

Hazard vulnerability analysis. Organizations must prepare Emergency Operations Plans (EOPs) to deal with any emergency that might occur. To develop an EOP, your organization needs to identify all emergencies that could occur within your facilities and community. Then leaders and staff must decide how likely each possible event is and what effect it would have on your facilities and community. This process, called a hazard vulnerability analysis (HVA), allows leaders to prioritize the emergency management plan and concentrate resources on the most likely and potentially serious events. The plan can then be tailored according to these priorities.

Phases of emergency management. For every emergency singled out in the HVA, you must consider the four essential phases of emergency management activities, which occur over time, in the following order:

- ***Mitigation:*** Actions taken in attempting to reduce the probably, severity, and/or impact of a potential emergency
- ***Preparedness:*** Actions taken to build capacity and identify resources that may be used if an emergency occurs
- ***Response:*** Actions taken when an emergency occurs
- ***Recovery:*** Actions taken to restore services after an emergency

Critical functions for emergency response. Several functions for an emergency response must be carefully planned due to their critical nature, particularly the following:

- ***Communication:*** Maintaining internal and external lines of communication with staff, community authorities, patients, media, suppliers, and other health care organizations
- ***Assets and resources:*** Acquiring and maintaining supplies, including water and fuel
- ***Safety and security:*** Maintaining a protected, safe environment for patients and workers, defining the roles of security agencies, controlling movements of people and traffic
- ***Staff responsibilities:*** Ensuring adequate staff and volunteers, identifying who does what and who reports to whom, providing training and support for staff (such as food and water, family care, and so on)
- ***Utilities management:*** Making sure that utilities (such as electricity) will be available during an emergency by having backups or alternate services
- ***Patient clinical and support activities:*** Delivering patient care (including that for vulnerable populations such as the elderly), documenting and tracking that care, taking care of mental and spiritual needs as well as personal hygiene and sanitation needs, evacuation as needed, and mortuary services

Emergency planning often focuses on hospital emergency departments and trauma centers, but when an emergency strikes the entire community, all health care organizations may be called upon. Therefore, all organizations should prepare to help with these critical functions, whether performing triage and urgent care of victims, sheltering community members or patients who have been evacuated from other facilities, or providing staff and/or supplies to other organizations.

Incident command structure. The critical functions of an emergency response should be anchored by an incident command structure (ICS). This system is essentially a command structure: it identifies the decision makers during an emergency and who will carry out those decisions. It doesn't need to be rigid; in fact, a flexible, adaptable ICS is more effective. This kind of approach, known as an "all-hazards" approach supports a general response capability that's sufficiently nimble to address a range of emergencies of different duration, scale, and cause.

Coordinated emergency management exercises. Being flexible doesn't mean you don't need to be prepared for specific types of emergencies. Like any plan, an emergency plan is only as good as the staff's ability to carry it out. This is why Joint Commission standards require organizations to run practical exercises on a regular basis. These are often based on specific scenarios. Plans should coordinate with relevant community resources, such as fire departments and other health care organizations.

Conversation Starters

Emergency Management

- *What types of emergencies and disasters are most likely to affect our community?*
- *Which community partners are important for us to work with to effectively manage emergencies?*
- *Do we have a process and structure for initiating an emergency management protocol?*
- *What hazards are we prepared to handle?*
- *Do we have any experience with these?*
- *Are there any emergency situations we need to work on developing more thorough plans to address?*

Hand-Off Communication

When a patient moves from an ambulatory care clinic to a hospital during an emergency, hand-off communication occurs. When a home care aide accompanies a patient moving to a nursing care center, hand-off communication occurs. When a nurse in an office-based surgery practice takes over a shift from another nurse, hand-off communication occurs. This kind of communication occurs whenever one or more health care workers transfers a patient's care responsibilities to one or more other health care workers or other caregivers. It's a frequent event—and a high-risk one. AHRQ reports that hand-offs have been linked to adverse events in almost every department of a hospital.[29] Many of these adverse events are the result of poor communication during patient hand-offs at transitions of care (when a patient is moved from one health care setting to another), such as transfer or discharge.[30]

Failures in hand-off communication. Failures in hand-off communication may result from the inability of the staff to construct an adequate shared picture of what's going on with the patient at the time of the hand-off as well as expectations and plans.[30] Common reasons for communication failures during hand-offs include the following[30]:

- Lack of formal supportive tools
- Variations in approaches
- Transactional in style rather than interactional
- Frequent interruptions

Standardizing a method. Although organizations recognize many of the reasons for failures, they continue to struggle with standardizing a method to address them. Some are conducted one-on-one, some in groups; some by phone, some in person; some using standardized tools, some without. Standardized hand-off protocols should address verbal, written, and electronic modes of communication. And they should consider how differing approaches among organizations with frequent hand-offs can coordinate most effectively. The Joint Commission Center for Transforming Healthcare offers the following solutions, which include standardization[31]:

- ***Standardization:***
  - Standardize the critical content (for example, patient history, treatment plan, key events).
  - Standardize forms, tools, or checklists to guide the discussion during hand-off communication.
  - Standardize education and coaching of staff on what constitutes a successful hand-off.

- ***Communication:*** Allow opportunities to ask questions during the hand-off (and exchange contact information in case there are questions later).
- ***Measurement:*** Collect and measure data to ensure the quality of hand-off communication.

Tools to help standardize hand-off communication. Just as they do for hand hygiene, the Center for Transforming Healthcare provides a Targeted Solutions Tool (TST) for hand-off communication. It's designed to help organizations discover their key reasons for failure and how to best address them in a standardized way. The TST can be accessed online at www.centerfortransforminghealthcare.org/tst_hoc.aspx. AHRQ also recommends standardizing hand-off protocols. It summarizes components of a successful organizationwide hand-off protocol using the mnemonic I-PASS[29]:

- Illness severity: a one-word summary of patient acuity ("stable," "watcher," or "unstable")
- Patient summary: a brief summary of the patient's diagnoses and treatment plan
- Action list: to-do items to be completed by the clinician receiving hand-off
- Situation awareness and contingency plans: directions to follow in case of changes in the patient's status, often in an "if-then" format
- Synthesis by receiver: an opportunity for the receiver to ask questions and confirm the plan of care

Call to Action
Hand-Off Communication

A board member must approach concerns with hand-off communication—and all other areas of quality and safety—with an open mind, curiosity, and gentle insistence on education, training, and data. You know that health care has complex systems, influenced by people, process, and technology. Hand-off communication involves many different people across shifts, departments, and organizations, and may involve several processes and converging technologies. The continued vigilance necessary to proactively prevent crises before they occur, particularly with such complex interactions, is a management and board challenge, but not an insurmountable one.

Organizations Helpful to Quality and Safety

In addition to the common areas of concern in quality and safety just covered, emerging areas that boards should consider learning more about include workplace violence, worker/staff fatigue, competency assessment, diagnostic errors, and diagnostic imaging. Note that these are not topics isolated to quality and safety in clinical care of the patient; they overlap and link to visitor and staff safety, widening the scope of impact for any risks. Indeed, quality and safety is a broad topic that touches almost every aspect of health care organizations and everyone involved in their operations. It can seem overwhelming in scope and importance. Luckily, there are a number of organizations that play a role in improving patient care and maximizing safety. This section will give you an overview of the organizations a board is likely to encounter—and consult—as it considers quality and safety.

The Joint Commission

The Joint Commission's mission is to continuously improve health care for the public. The nonprofit organization collaborates with other stakeholders to evaluate health care organizations and inspire them to excel in providing the safest possible care at the best value. Its comprehensive Web portal (www.jointcommission.org) offers a wealth of useful information and resources that support its programs and services. Chapter 2 will provide more information on those Joint Commission services important to board members and their roles in quality and safety.

Programs and services. To accomplish its mission, The Joint Commission provides the following programs and services:

- ***Accreditation and certification:*** This includes the establishment of standards as well as patient-centered on-site evaluations (surveys) for every care setting across the continuum and every clinical diagnosis.
- ***Performance measurement:*** A service for hospitals, this is done through the ORYX® initiative and involves the development and implementation of standardized core measures ("accountability measures") that focus on the importance of the relationship of reliable care processes to patient outcomes.
- ***Patient safety efforts:*** These efforts include the formation of National Patient Safety Goals and the development of a "Patient Safety Systems" chapter in the standards manuals, which provides the basics of patient safety science.
- ***Sentinel event review process:*** A *sentinel event* is a type of adverse event resulting in a patient's death, permanent harm, or severe temporary harm that isn't primarily related to the natural course of a patient's illness or an underlying condition. The term *sentinel* is used because it signals the need for immediate

investigation and response. Review of these events is performed by uniquely qualified and certified safety specialists. They review the sentinel events with accredited organizations and maintain the Sentinel Event Database, disseminating shared learnings through *Sentinel Event Alerts* and the monthly *Quick Safety* newsletter, which are publicly available on the Joint Commission website.

- ***The Center for Transforming Healthcare:*** This arm of The Joint Commission enterprise is focused on finding solutions for health care's most intractable problems and is devoted to moving health care toward high reliability (*see* Chapter 2).
- ***Gold Seal of Approval®:*** Via its Quality Check® website at www.qualitycheck.org, the public and the health care field can search by organization, service, state, city, or zip code to see which organizations have achieved Joint Commission accreditation and certification, marked by the Gold Seal of Approval.
- ***Public policy initiatives:*** These address public policy topics such as nurse staffing, emergency preparedness, emergency department overcrowding, pay-for-performance programs, organ donation, prevention of workplace violence, and health care professionals' education
- ***Innovative solutions:*** Through its subsidiary, Joint Commission Resources, The Joint Commission provides consulting, electronic products, publications, and education to help health care organizations learn about quality and safety issues and find innovative solutions to compliance problems.

Centers for Medicare & Medicaid Services

The Centers for Medicare & Medicaid Services (CMS) has a significant influence on health care quality assurance and PI. The Medicare program reimbursed health care providers for nearly $600 billion in services in fiscal year 2014.[32] Reimbursement, though, is dependent on the organization meeting CMS standards of care, commonly known as Conditions of Participation (CoPs) and Conditions for Coverage (CfCs), depending on the setting of care. And, as a result of the ACA, CMS does not reimburse hospitals for serious reportable events, such as wrong-site surgeries, pressure ulcers, transfusion with the wrong blood type, and other HACs. *See* Sidebar 1-2, page 48, for a list of HACs that CMS does not reimburse.

HACs and HCACs. Note that the term *health care–acquired condition* (HCAC) has entered the general parlance of health care content. It's a term used by CMS under the umbrella term *provider preventable conditions* (PPCs). It relates to a rule that prevents Medicaid payments for PPCs in inpatient settings and to patients eligible for both Medicare and Medicaid programs. The list of nonreimburseable Medicaid HCACs is the same as the HAC Medicare list for now. Medicaid also has another category of PPCs that apply to any health care setting.[33]

SIDEBAR 1-2

Nonreimburseable HACs/HCACs

Following is the list of current hospital-acquired conditions (HACs)/health care–acquired conditions (HCACs) for which Centers for Medicare & Medicaid Services will not reimburse inpatient health care organizations:

- Foreign object retained after surgery
- Air embolism (when air enters a vein or artery)
- Blood incompatibility (when two different blood types are mixed)
- Stage III and IV pressure ulcers (serious sores on the skin and underlying tissues that result from being in the same position for a long time)
- Falls and trauma:
  - Fractures
  - Dislocations
  - Intracranial injuries (injuries to the brain from an external source)
  - Crushing injuries
  - Burns
- Other injuries (related to the fall or subsequent care):
  - Manifestations of poor glycemic control
  - Diabetic ketoacidosis (preventable high blood sugars causing a chemical imbalance)
  - Nonketotic hyperosmolar coma (coma state due to severe dehydration caused by seriously high blood sugar)
  - Hypoglycemic coma (coma state due to seriously low blood sugar)
  - Secondary diabetes with ketoacidosis (severely high blood sugar that occurs when a patient's diabetes is the result of another medical condition)
  - Secondary diabetes with hyperosmolarity (severe dehydration that occurs when the patient's diabetes is the result of another medical condition)
- Catheter-associated urinary tract infection (infection in bladder and kidneys due to a catheter)
- Vascular (central line) catheter–associated infection (infection in bloodstream due to an IV catheter)
- Surgical site infection after the following procedures:
  - Coronary artery bypass graft mediastinitis (an infection in the chest cavity due to a particular kind of surgery that improves blood flow to the heart)
  - Bariatric surgery:
    - Laparoscopic gastric bypass (minimally invasive procedure that creates a gastric pouch to bypass part of the digestive process)
    - Gastroenterostomy (procedure that creates an opening between the stomach and small intestine to allow food to move through the digestive tract more easily)

    - Laparoscopic gastric restrictive surgery (minimally invasive procedure that restricts food intake, such as gastric banding or "stomach stapling")
  - Orthopedic surgery:
    - Spine
    - Neck
    - Shoulder
    - Elbow
  - Cardiac implantable electronic device (pacemaker, defibrillator, ventricular assisted device)
- Deep vein thrombosis (blood clots in deep veins)/pulmonary embolism (blockage in an artery in a lung) after the following:
  - Total knee replacement
  - Hip replacement
  - Latrogenic pneumothorax with venous catheterization (collapsed lung caused by a medical procedure involving insertion of a central venous catheter)

Source: Adapted from Centers for Medicare & Medicaid Services. Hospital-Acquired Conditions. (Updated: Aug 19, 2015.) Accessed Aug 26, 2016. https://www.cms.gov/medicare/medicare-fee-for-service-payment/hospitalacqcond/hospital-acquired_conditions.html.

CMS incentives for quality care. Since the ACA, CMS also strives to link Medicare reimbursement with the quality of care, not just the quantity of services provided. Formerly, payments were based on how many times an organization performed a service. In other words, the legislation now has CMS shift a portion of the reimbursement to a payment-for-quality system, rather than a strict payment-for-volume system. As described earlier in this chapter, the VBP system uses existing health care organization quality data reporting structures to incentivize high-quality care. For example, for hospitals, the Hospital Compare consumer-oriented website (www.medicare.gov/hospitalcompare/) provides a summary of hospitals' performance in the following areas[34]:

- Patient experience
- Timely and effective care, based on a selection of process and outcome measures
- Complications and serious reportable events
- Readmissions and deaths, compared to national rates
- Use of medical imaging
- Payment and value of care for particular conditions, compared to the national average

Hospitals are eligible for a payment incentive only if they report their performance data to CMS for Hospital Compare.

Quality improvement organizations (QIOs). Working under the direction of CMS are groups of health quality experts, clinicians, and consumers organized to improve the care delivered to people with Medicare. These groups are known as quality improvement organizations (QIOs). They assist Medicare providers with quality improvement and review quality concerns for the protection of beneficiaries and the Medicare Trust Fund.

CMS and Joint Commission alignment. The Joint Commission works closely with CMS to align its requirements for performance measures (such as the "accountability measure" mentioned above), especially as CMS has advanced toward "e-measures," or electronic clinical quality measures (eCQMs), rather than the classic chart-abstracted measures. The Joint Commission also has and enforces standards and a survey process that meet or exceed the Medicare CoPs. As CMS updates its Medicare CoPs, The Joint Commission updates relevant standards and elements of performance (EPs) in an effort to align expectations and minimize data collection by eliminating redundancies. This information is available as a crosswalk between CMS and Joint Commission requirements in certain Joint Commission Resources products. An understanding of the alignment and crosswalk is instrumental in seeking deemed status.

Deemed status. Certain patient care organizations (hospitals, critical access hospitals, ambulatory surgery centers, advanced diagnostic imaging locations, home health, hospice, durable medical equipment, and laboratories) must have CMS certification—or they can seek "deemed status" provided by an accrediting organization or state surveys. This means that health care organizations may elect to use Joint Commission accreditation as proof of meeting CMS requirements for reimbursement. The Joint Commission is the only accrediting organization that's authorized as having deeming authority for *all* these clinical settings (where deeming status is relevant).

More information on CMS can be found on its website at www.cms.gov/.

Conversation Starters
Centers for Medicare & Medicaid Services

- *How much reimbursement have we lost as a result of HACs/HCACs?*
- *What are we doing to prevent this in the future?*
- *How does our organization rate in the VBP data collected and shared on the CMS and Hospital Compare websites?*
- *Are we seeking or have we attained deemed status?*
- *Has CMS come in and done a look-behind survey?*

Institute for Healthcare Improvement

The Institute for Healthcare Improvement (IHI) began decades ago as an organization dedicated to identification of and education on best practices in health care. It has since evolved beyond that narrower focus, and now approaches health care as a "complete social, geopolitical enterprise," focusing on the following key areas[35]:

- Improvement capability
- Person- and family-centered care
- Patient safety
- Quality, cost, and value
- Triple Aim for populations (simultaneously improve care, improve population health, and reduce per capita costs)

100 Million Healthier Lives campaign. Chief among IHI's strategic initiatives is the 100 Million Healthier Lives campaign, which is striving for 100 million people living healthier lives by 2020. This initiative identifies innovative, effective health care models around the world, engaging industry leaders to make those models applicable on a larger scale. The program focuses on the following core strategies:

- Creating health care systems that are good at health and good at care
- Bridging health care, community, public health, and social services
- Creating healthy communities
- Empowering individuals through peer-to-peer support networks
- Creating underlying conditions that support better care, such as new payment structures and policy changes
- Developing new mind-sets about partnerships, collaboration, and "servant leadership" that support better care

Collaboration is the key tool the 100 Million Healthier Lives initiative uses to blend these priorities into cohesive systematic changes. Dozens of organizations have joined with IHI to lead the campaign, including community health and youth organizations; health care delivery systems; universities, colleges, and other learning institutions; federal, state, and local governmental agencies; philanthropic organizations; professional groups; and consulting and research organizations. In the United States, participating leaders include the CDC, Centers for Medicare & Medicaid Innovation, HHS, American Academy of Nursing, and American Psychological Association.[36]

IHI leadership resources. IHI has an online library of resources, including tools, publications, case studies, and audio/video presentations, designed to help organizations and their leadership with improvement efforts. IHI believes that highly engaged leadership is essential to high-quality care, so it has created a special collection of resources, available online, to help boards improve their effectiveness in this area: www.ihi.org/Topics/GovernanceLeadership.

Health and Medicine Division of the National Academies of Sciences, Engineering, and Medicine

The Health and Medicine Division (HMD) of the National Academies of Sciences, Engineering, and Medicine (the Academies) is a private, nonprofit organization dedicated to supporting informed decision making in the governmental and private sectors. Formerly known as the Institute of Medicine (IOM), it provides reliable information through scientific studies, consensus committees, and other cross-disciplinary forums. Among its work are two classic reports.

Two classic health care reports. The following reports issued by the Academies' Committee on the Quality of Health Care in America laid the groundwork for current thinking on hospital PI:

- ***To Err Is Human: Building a Safer Health System (1999):*** This report outlines a comprehensive strategy for reducing preventable medical adverse events. The strategy engaged health care providers, governmental agencies, industry stakeholders, and consumers to achieve a minimum goal of 50% reduction in errors during the subsequent five years.[37]
- ***Crossing the Quality Chasm:*** A New Health System for the 21st Century (2001): This follow-up to the 1999 report addresses restructuring the health care system as a whole (including delivery and payment mechanisms) to provide better patient care and to make the best use of available resources. The proposed focus is on chronic conditions, which demand more resources than acute

episodic care, and the goal for all proposed changes is to have care that meets the following six "Aims for Improvement"[38]:

- Safety
- Effectiveness
- Patient-centeredness
- Timeliness
- Efficiency
- Equity

Crossing the Quality Chasm asserts that the individual patient experience should be the guide for assessing the quality of hospitals, care delivery, and health care policies. And it highlights six challenges for health care organizations that are still applicable today[38]:

- Redesigning care processes to better serve chronically ill patients across settings, among clinicians, and over time
- Using information technology to automate clinical information and make it accessible to patients and clinicians
- Managing the ever-increasing advances in methods/techniques and ensuring that health care professionals are competent to use them
- Coordinating care across conditions, settings, and services over time
- Working to build more effective multidisciplinary teams
- Incorporating process and outcome measures into day-to-day activities

Impact of the reports. These publications have helped organizational leaders, health care providers, patients, and policy makers focus more on safety. And that has helped the industry more clearly identify the critical factors in quality and safety, most of which have been addressed in this chapter: transparency, communication, teamwork, patient engagement, organizational safety culture, and human factors engineering (the study of how people perform tasks). The impact of these reports is also seen in the use of evidence-based care, the recognition of the link between increased safety and greater quality and value, and the incorporation of patient safety into health care education and training curricula.[39]

Progress in improving quality and safety, however, has not met expectations. Why? Both reports emphasize that the majority of errors result from faulty systems and processes rather than from the actions of specific individuals. They conclude that the only way to reduce errors is to shift the focus to change the systems and processes themselves. Due in part to the unexpected complexity of safety issues, however, improvement efforts have followed a haphazard issue-based approach instead of making fundamental changes to the underlying systems and processes. Also, the urgency that swept through health care in the wake of these reports has diminished in the past 15 years since they were published, putting patient safety again "in the backseat."[39]

A total systems approach. Going forward, the HMD recognizes that health care must continue to move away from an approach that aims to improve specific safety metrics, which has shown mixed results and puts further stress on the organizations and care providers. Instead, it recommends that organizations push toward that total systems approach in which safety is prioritized uniformly across the organization. To do this, the HMD recommends the following[39]:

- Ensure that leaders establish and sustain a safety culture.
- Create a centralized, coordinated oversight of patient safety.
- Create a common set of safety-related metrics that reflect meaningful outcomes.
- Increase funding for patient safety research.
- Prioritize safety across the health care continuum.
- Support the health care workforce.
- Partner with patients and families for the safest care.
- Ensure that technology is safe and used to further improve safety.

Prioritizing safety in every aspect of health care is a central component of the high reliability approach, which will be addressed in greater detail in Chapter 2. Involving leaders, including the board, in an integrated way, will be discussed in Chapter 3.

An important report on nursing. *The Future of Nursing: Leading Change, Advancing Health* (2011) is another groundbreaking report. A joint effort of the Robert Wood Johnson Foundation and the Academies, this report focuses on increasing the effectiveness of the United States' largest population of health care workers: registered professional nurses. This publication describes eight strategies to optimize registered nurses' practice, consistent with the goals of the IHI Triple Aim, cited above. These are as follows[40]:

- Remove scope-of-practice barriers so advanced practice registered nurses are able to practice to the full extent of their education and training.
- Expand opportunities for nurses to lead and manage collaborative improvement efforts.
- Implement nurse residency programs to facilitate transitions into or between clinical practice areas
- Increase the proportion of nurses with a baccalaureate degree, with a goal of 80% by 2020.

- Double the number of nurses with a doctorate by 2020.
- Ensure that nurses engage in lifelong learning.
- Prepare and enable nurses to lead changes in health care.
- Build an infrastructure for the collection and analysis of health care workforce data.

More information on the HMD can be found on the Academies website at www.nationalacademies.org/hmd/.

National Patient Safety Foundation

Founded in 1997, the National Patient Safety Foundation (NPSF) is an independent, not-for-profit organization that aims to engage key stakeholders to advance patient safety, promote health care worker safety, and disseminate strategies to prevent harm. NPSF focuses on the safety of both patients and staff—a feature that differentiates this organization's efforts from others.

The Lucian Leape Institute. One of NPSF's central components is the Lucian Leape Institute. This is a "think tank" devoted to studying key safety topics, and to date has disseminated learnings on five fundamental concepts critical to achieving meaningful improvements in safety systems:

- Transparency
- Care integration
- Patient/family/consumer engagement
- Workforce safety, including joy and meaning in health care work
- Medical education reform

NPSF events, groups, and programs. Other NPSF initiatives center on an annual "Patient Safety Awareness Week," an event that brings together health care providers, consumers, associations, and public and private companies to focus on the importance of harm prevention. Additional NPSF components include individual and corporate memberships in groups devoted to patient safety as well as certification programs for individuals working in the quality and safety field across many settings and disciplines.

More information on NPSF can be found on its website at www.npsf.org.

National Quality Forum

The National Quality Forum (NQF) is a not-for-profit, national membership organization that aims to improve health and health care quality through measurement and reporting. Its members are invited from many areas of health care, and its stakeholders include the following:

- Providers
- Insurers
- Employers
- Consumer groups
- Professional associations
- Accrediting bodies (including The Joint Commission)
- Researchers
- Labor unions

NQF brings together leaders in these public- and private-sector organizations to create national standards and priorities in health care: a "single language" for discussing health care quality and efficiency in the United States.[41] NQF has, for example, endorsed a set of safe practices (or voluntary consensus standards) that clinical care settings can use to reduce the risk of harm to patients.

National Quality Strategy and the ACA. NQF bases much of its work on the National Quality Strategy (NQS), which is a fundamental component of the ACA. The NQS acts as a national blueprint for improving quality and safety in health care. It sets goals and describes a strategic plan for achieving them. These goals address the quality and safety issues that affect most Americans[42]:

- Patient safety
- Health and well-being
- Prevention and treatment of leading causes of mortality
- Person- and family-centered care
- Effective communication and care coordination
- Affordable care

In addition, NQF addresses the following:

- Palliative and end-of-life care
- Disparities in health care related to socioeconomic, demographic, or cultural factors
- HIT as it relates to safety, care coordination, data reporting, and other issues

Serious reportable events list. NQF maintains a list of serious reportable events (SREs) in health care. Currently, 29 adverse events are considered to be serious, largely preventable, and of concern to both the public and health care providers. Many states use NQF's list as the basis for their own reporting systems, as described earlier in this chapter. NQF divides these events into the following areas:

- Surgical or invasive procedure events
- Product or device events
- Patient protection events
- Care management events
- Environmental events
- Radiologic events
- Potential criminal events

To learn more about NQF, visit its website at www.qualityforum.org.

Agency for Healthcare Research and Quality

The Agency for Healthcare Research and Quality (AHRQ) is part of HHS. Its focus is to produce reliable evidence and work to make that evidence understood so that health care providers and policy makers can make informed decisions about health care improvement.

In addition to funding and publishing research and statistical data related to health care quality and safety, AHRQ has developed initiatives based in large part on the *To Err Is Human* report discussed above. Some of these initiatives include the following:

- ***Re-Engineered Discharge (RED):*** A structured process and set of tools to help hospitals design and communicate effective discharge plans to reduce patients' hospital readmissions
- ***Comprehensive Unit-based Safety Program (CUSP):*** A training module designed to prevent central line– and catheter-associated urinary tract infections
- ***TeamSTEPPS®:*** A training program, developed in conjunction with the US Department of Defense and promoted in partnership with CMS, for health care professionals to develop their communication and teamwork skills as a means of improving patient safety

And, as noted in the earlier discussion on safety culture, AHRQ also sponsored the development of several setting-specific safety culture surveys that many organizations use to assess and improve their patient safety culture.

AHRQ partnering with The Joint Commission. The Joint Commission uses AHRQ data to inform its accreditation standards and as a guide for a number of recommendations on numerous topics. For example, The Joint Commission's

Primary Care Medical Home (PCMH) model is based on AHRQ's definition of a medical home. Also, AHRQ has provided funds for the development of Joint Commission tools and resources, such as an online learning module related to infection prevention and control in nursing care center facilities. The Joint Commission is just one of many organizations that partners with AHRQ.

AHRQ's research findings, statistical reports, and more can be accessed online at www.ahrq.gov.

The Leapfrog Group

The Leapfrog Group focuses on the principle that its members' collective purchasing power can be leveraged to improve the safety, quality, and affordability of health care. Its membership encompasses large private and public health care purchasers, including Fortune 500 companies.

Leapfrog Hospital Survey and Hospital Recognition Program. The Leapfrog Hospital Recognition Program measures performance through data submitted via its annual Leapfrog Hospital Survey. The survey collects self-reported performance data based on national quality and safety measures, many of which are endorsed by or complimentary to Joint Commission, NQF, and CMS. Leapfrog assesses performance measures in the following areas[43]:

- CPOE
- Evidence-based hospital referral
- Maternity care
- ICU physician staffing
- NQF's Safe Practices
- Managing serious errors
- BCMA
- Resource utilization for common acute conditions

Leapfrog's Hospital Safety Score gives each hospital a letter grade rating of how well it protects patients from HACs such as infections, injuries, and medical errors. The grade is based on the self-reported data from the Leapfrog Hospital Survey and data from sources such as CMS and the American Hospital Association.

The survey and recognition program initiatives are rooted in the concept that transparency is critical to motivating improvement. If health care consumers—patients and employers—can see hospitals' quality and safety data, they can "shop around" for the best care. Hospitals can attract these consumers by having excellent quality and safety.

Quality, safety, and value. In addition to quality and safety, Leapfrog focuses on value. One tool it has developed to assess health care value is the Hidden Surcharge Calculator. Employers can also use a facility's Hospital Safety Score in conjunction with its own claims data to estimate the amount they are paying per admission for hospital errors. This can help the employer save costs by directing their employees to hospitals with a higher safety record. This also encourages hospitals to improve their performance in order to attract or retain those health care consumers.[44]

For more information on the Leapfrog Group, visit their website at www.leapfroggroup.org.

Call to Action
Organizations Helpful to Quality and Safety

As you and other board members strive to understand the complexity of quality and safety in health care, accessing and learning about the key initiatives and resources from each of these quality and safety organizations can be helpful. A particular emphasis on goals for your own board's education, aligned with the strategic goals of the health care organization you serve, can help direct which of the highlighted organizations are most important to more deeply explore and understand. New board members will want to assess how each organization's work can complement those quality and safety strategies important to your own situation.

The Next Step

As this chapter has explained, quality and safety must be a priority in health care organizations: There are board responsibilities for quality and safety, factors affecting quality and safety, common areas of concern in quality and safety, and organizations helpful to quality and safety. Leadership, including the board, must be aware of all this and must actively foster an environment in which related challenges can be overcome. Chapter 2 will explore how The Joint Commission supports those efforts through its accreditation and certification processes, and describes Joint Commission services that can help an organization achieve and maintain that quality and safety.

REFERENCES

1. Combes JR, Totten MK, Prybil LD. Helping boards achieve and demonstrate accountability: Taking responsibility to new levels. *Healthc Exec.* 2014 May–Jun;29(3):76, 78.
2. Belmont E, et al. A new quality compass: Hospital boards' increased role under the Affordable Care Act. *Health Aff (Millwood).* 2011 Jul;30(7):1282–1289. Accessed Aug 22, 2016. http://content.healthaffairs.org/content/30/7/1282.long.
3. Hanlon C, et al. *2014 Guide to State Adverse Event Reporting Systems.* Washington, DC: National Academy for State Health Policy, 2015. Accessed Aug 22, 2016. http://www.nashp.org/sites/default/files/2014_Guide_to_State_Adverse_Event_Reporting_Systems.pdf.
4. National Quality Forum (NQF). *Serious Reportable Events in Healthcare—2011 Update: A Consensus Report.* Washington, DC: NQF, 2011. Accessed Aug 22, 2016. http://www.qualityforum.org/WorkArea/linkit.aspx?LinkIdentifier=id&ItemID=69573.
5. Agency for Healthcare Research and Quality. The Role of the Patient in Safety. (Updated: Jul 2016.) Accessed Aug 22, 2016. https://psnet.ahrq.gov/primers/primer/17/the-role-of-the-patient-in-safety.
6. US Department of Health and Human Services. The Affordable Care Act Is Working. Jun 24, 2015. Accessed Aug 25, 2016. http://www.hhs.gov/healthcare/facts-and-features/fact-sheets/aca-is-working/index.html.
7. Medicare.gov. Linking Quality to Payment. Accessed Aug 25, 2016. https://www.medicare.gov/hospitalcompare/linking-quality-to-payment.html?AspxAutoDetectCookieSupport=1.
8. US Department of Health and Human Services. Press Release: New HHS Data Show Quality Improvements Saved 15,000 Lives and $4 Billion in Health Spending. May 7, 2015. Accessed Aug 25, 2016. http://www.hhs.gov/about/news/2014/05/07/new-hhs-data-show-quality-improvements-saved-15000-lives-and-4-billion-in-health-spending.html.
9. US Department of Health and Human Services. Press Release: Efforts to Improve Patient Safety Result in 1.3 Million Fewer Patient Harms, 50,000 Lives Saved and $12 Billion in Health Spending Avoided. Dec 2, 2014. Accessed Aug 25, 2016. http://www.hhs.gov/about/news/2014/12/02/efforts-improve-patient-safety-result-1-3-million-fewer-patient-harms-50000-lives-saved-and-12-billion-in-health-spending-avoided.html.
10. Centers for Medicare & Medicaid Services. Bundled Payments for Care Improvement (BPCI) Initiative: General Information. (Updated: Jul 19, 2016.) Accessed Aug 25, 2016. https://innovation.cms.gov/initiatives/bundled-payments/.
11. Internal Revenue Service. New Requirements for 501(c)(3) Hospitals Under the Affordable Care Act. (Updated: Jul 29, 2016.) Accessed Aug 25, 2016. https://www.irs.gov/charities-non-profits/charitable-organizations/new-requirements-for-501c3-hospitals-under-the-affordable-care-act.

12. Center for Health Design. The Role of the Physical Environment in the 21st Century: A Once-in-a-Lifetime Opportunity. Ulrich R, et al. Sep 2004. Accessed Aug 25, 2016. https://www.healthdesign.org/sites/default/files/Role%20Physical%20Environ%20in%20the%2021st%20Century%20Hospital_0.pdf.
13. Centers for Disease Control and Prevention. Healthcare-Associated Infections: HAI Data and Statistics. (Updated: Mar 2, 2016.) Accessed Aug 25, 2016. http://www.cdc.gov/HAI/surveillance/.
14. Centers for Disease Control and Prevention. Influenza (Flu): Influenza Vaccination Information for Health Care Workers. (Updated: Aug 25, 2016.) Accessed Aug 26, 2016. http://www.cdc.gov/flu/healthcareworkers.htm.
15. American Association of Colleges of Nursing. Nursing Shortage. (Updated: Apr 24, 2014.) Accessed Aug 26, 2016. http://www.aacn.nche.edu/media-relations/fact-sheets/nursing-shortage.
16. Kalisch BJ, Xie B. Errors of omission: Missed nursing care. West J Nurs Res. 2014 Apr 29;36(7):875–890.
17. Duffin C. Increase in nurse numbers linked to better patient survival rates in ICU. Nurs Stand. 2014 Apr 16–22;28(33):10.
18. Frost SA, Alexandrou E. Higher nurse staffing levels associated with reductions in unplanned readmissions to intensive care or operating theatre, and in postoperative in-hospital mortality in heart surgery patients. *Evid Based Nurs*. 2013 Apr;16(2):62–3.
19. McHugh MD, Ma C. Hospital nursing and 30-day readmissions among Medicare patients with heart failure, acute myocardial infarction, and pneumonia. Med Care. 2013 Jan;51(1):52–59.
20. Mansur JM. Medication safety systems and the important role of pharmacists. *Drugs Aging*. 2016 Mar;33(3):213–221.
21. Sigma Theta Tau International. Nurse-Patient Assignments: Moving Beyond Nurse-Patient Ratios for Better Patient, Staff, and Organizational Outcomes. Allen SB. Nov 8, 2015. Abstract. Accessed Aug 26, 2016. https://stti.confex.com/stti/bc43/webprogram/Paper74725.html.
22. Nursing Solutions, Inc. 2016 National Healthcare Retention & RN Staffing Report. Mar 2016. Accessed Aug 26, 2016. http://www.nsinursingsolutions.com/files/assets/library/retention-institute/NationalHealthcareRNRetentionReport2016.pdf.
23. Press Ganey. *Nursing Special Report: The Influence of Nurse Work Environment on Patient, Payment and Nurse Outcomes in Acute Care Settings*. South Bend, IN: Press Ganey Associates, 2015.
24. The Joint Commission, Office of Quality and Patient Safety. *Sentinel Event Data: Root Causes by Event Type: 2004–2015*. Oak Brook, IL: The Joint Commission, 2016.
25. Grissinger M. Medication errors involving overrides of healthcare technology. *Pennsylvania Patient Safety Advisory*. 2015 Dec;12(4):141–148.
26. Khanna R, Yen T. Computerized physician order entry: Promise, perils, and experience. *Neurohospitalist*. 2014 Jan;4(1):26–33.
27. Rack LL, Dudjak LA, Wolf GA. Study of nurse workarounds in a hospital using bar code medication administration system. *J Nurs Care Qual*. 2012 Jul–Sep;27(3):232–239.
28. The Joint Commission. Safe use of health information technology. Sentinel Event Alert. 2015 Mar 31;(54):1–6. Accessed Aug 26, 2015. http://www.jointcommission.org/assets/1/18/SEA_54.pdf.
29. Agency for Healthcare Research and Quality. Handoffs and Signouts. (Updated: Jul 2016.) Accessed Aug 26, 2016. https://psnet.ahrq.gov/primers/primer/9.
30. The Joint Commission: *Improving Hand-Off Communication*. Oak Brook, IL: Joint Commission Resources, 2007.

31. Joint Commission Center for Transforming Healthcare. Facts About the Hand-Off Communications Project. Accessed Aug 26, 2016. http://www.centerfortransforminghealthcare.org/assets/4/6/CTH_HOC_Fact_Sheet.pdf.

32. US Department of Health and Human Services. 2014 CMS Statistics. Aug 2014. Accessed Aug 26, 2016. https://www.cms.gov/Research-Statistics-Data-and-Systems/Statistics-Trends-and-Reports/CMS-Statistics-Reference-Booklet/Downloads/CMS_Stats_2014_final.pdf#tableiii5.

33. American College of Emergency Physicians. Health Care-Acquired & Provider Preventable Conditions FAQ. (Updated: Feb 17, 2016.) Accessed Aug 26, 2016. https://www.acep.org/Clinical—Practice-Management/Health-Care-Acquired—Provider-Preventable-Conditions-FAQ/.

34. Medicare.gov. About Hospital Compare: What Information Can I Get About Hospitals? Accessed Aug 26, 2016. https://www.medicare.gov/hospitalcompare/About/Hospital-Info.html.

35. Institute for Healthcare Improvement. About Us: About IHI. Accessed Aug 26, 2016. http://www.ihi.org/about/Pages/default.aspx.

36. 100 Million Healthier Lives. Home page. Accessed Aug 26, 2016. http://www.100mlives.org/.

37. Institute of Medicine. *To Err Is Human: Building a Safer Health System*. Washington, DC: National Academy Press, 2000.

38. Institute of Medicine. Crossing the Quality Chasm: *A New Health System for the 21st Century*. Washington, DC: National Academy Press, 2001.

39. National Patient Safety Foundation (NPSF). *Free from Harm: Accelerating Patient Safety Improvement Fifteen Years After To Err Is Human*. Boston: NPSF, 2015.

40. Institute of Medicine. *The Future of Nursing: Leading Change, Advancing Health*. Washington, DC: National Academies Press, 2011.

41. National Quality Forum. NQF's Mission and Vision. Accessed Aug 26, 2016. http://www.qualityforum.org/About_NQF/Mission_and_Vision.aspx.

42. National Quality Forum. Improving Health and Healthcare. Accessed Aug 26, 2016. http://www.qualityforum.org/Topics/Improving_Health_and_Healthcare.aspx.

43. The Leapfrog Group. Welcome to the 2016 Leapfrog Group Hospital Survey. Accessed Aug 26, 2016. http://www.leapfroggroup.org/survey-materials.

44. The Leapfrog Group. Value Tools. Accessed Aug 26, 2016. http://www.leapfroggroup.org/employers-purchasers/value-tools.

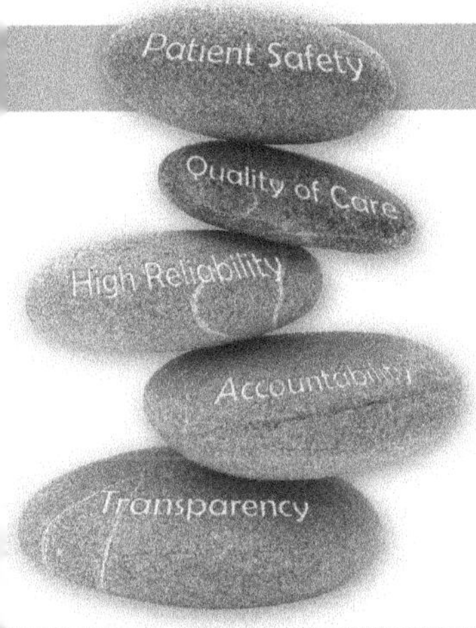

Chapter 2

Introduction to The Joint Commission

As a board member, you may be most familiar with The Joint Commission as an accrediting body for health care organizations. But The Joint Commission is actually an enterprise composed of the following not-for-profit companies, which work together to help organizations like yours improve health care quality and safety by providing a range of programs and services:

- ***The Joint Commission:*** The oldest and largest accrediting body in health care in the United States (*see* www.jointcommission.org)
- ***Joint Commission Resources:*** A subsidiary of The Joint Commission that offers health care education, publications, electronic products, and consultation services (*see* www.jcrinc.com)
- ***Joint Commission International:*** A division of Joint Commission Resources that serves as a quality and safety accreditor in more than 90 countries (*see* www.jointcommissioninternational.org)
- ***The Joint Commission Center for Transforming Healthcare:*** An organization that targets the most critical quality and safety problems and delivers practical solutions (*see* www.centerfortransforminghealthcare.org)

This chapter will help you understand what you need to know about The Joint Commission enterprise and its work by providing an introduction to the following:

Joint Commission Accreditation
- Accreditation as a Proven Approach
- Accreditation as a Value Equation
- Accreditation Requirements
- Accreditation Requirements for the Board

The Joint Commission Accreditation Process
- The On-Site Survey
- The Accreditation Decision
- Tracer Methodology
- Risk Classification and the SAFER™ Matrix
- Continuous Compliance
- Quality Reports® and Quality Check®

The Joint Commission and Measurement
- Accountability Measures
- The ORYX® Initiative
- Library of Other Measures
- Alignment with CMS Measures

The Joint Commission and Patient Safety
- Learning from Patient Safety Events
- Leadership in Patient Safety
- Reporting and Responding to Patient Safety Events
- Risk Management to Prevent Patient Safety Events
- The Patient's Role in Patient Safety

The Joint Commission and High Reliability
- Framework of Changes for the Journey to High Reliability
- High Reliability Principles
- High Reliability: Looking Forward
- The Next Step

Joint Commission Accreditation

The Joint Commission accredits most hospitals in the United States, and started out as The Joint Commission on Accreditation of Hospitals (JCAHO). But its market share has expanded, and today nearly 22,000 health care organizations and programs nationwide use Joint Commission requirements and performance measures to guide how they administer care and continuously improve performance. They work hard to earn and maintain the distinction of being Joint Commission–accredited. Why? What does it mean to be accredited? And what kinds of organizations and programs can earn accreditation?

Accreditation vs. certification. Joint Commission accreditation can be earned by many types of health care organizations, including hospitals, physician's offices, nursing homes, office-based surgery centers, behavioral health treatment facilities, and providers of home care services. Certification is earned by programs or services that may be based within or associated with a health care organization. For example, a Joint Commission–accredited medical center can have Joint Commission–certified programs or services within orthopedics. In this chapter, unless otherwise clarified, the term *accreditation* will be used to embrace the overall concept, which may include certification. Table 2-1 on page 66 lists the various accreditation and certification options available through The Joint Commission.

Accreditation as a Proven Approach

Accreditation isn't a simple evaluation or business transaction. The Joint Commission develops an interactive working relationship with each of its accredited organizations and programs. This relationship is reflected in The Joint Commission's mission, which is "to continuously improve health care for the public, in collaboration with other stakeholders, by evaluating health care organizations and inspiring them to excel in providing safe and effective care of the highest quality and value."[1]

Accreditation of organizations helps to fulfill that mission: The entire purpose of Joint Commission accreditation is to support organizations in the delivery of high-quality patient care and safety. Through accreditation your organization can develop the critical infrastructure for quality and safety, allowing it to improve performance over time. This is because accreditation helps health care organizations standardize their systems and processes of care. Standardization leads to fewer variations, which can result in more positive outcomes as well as decreased costs and minimized risks. As health care organizations learn about the value of standardization through accreditation to improve quality and safety, they're primed to develop into more highly reliable organizations (*see* page 96).

Resources for learning and development. The Joint Commission's commitment to quality and safety learning and development for organizations is demonstrated by the number and scope of resources available as complimentary tools for accredited organizations. One of the most valuable is the Core Measure Solution Exchange®, a social media site exclusively for accredited hospitals where they can learn from each other's solutions to improve their core measure performance. This resource is especially important under the reforms of the Affordable Care Act (ACA), which tie reimbursement to performance on these and other

TABLE 2-1: Joint Commission Accreditation and Certification Programs

This table lists the accreditation and certification programs The Joint Commission offers. More information on each is available on The Joint Commission website: www.jointcommission.org.

Accreditation Programs	Certification Programs
• **Ambulatory Health Care:** Includes ambulatory surgery centers, advanced diagnostic imaging, group practices, sleep labs, telemedicine, and office-based surgery practices, among others • **Behavioral Health Care:** Encompasses a wide range of services and programs, including addiction services and opioid treatment programs • **Critical Access Hospitals:** Applies to hospitals with 25 beds or less, that keep patients hospitalized for 96 hours or less, and have received appropriate authorization from the state office of rural health • **Home Care:** Includes home health, durable medical equipment, pharmacy, and hospice services • **Hospitals:** Includes general, academic medical centers, psychiatric, children's, specialty (such as cancer hospitals), surgical, long term acute care, and rehabilitation hospitals • **Nursing Care Centers:** Also known as long term care; skilled nursing facilities • **Laboratory:** Includes both independent and freestanding laboratories	• **Advanced Certification in Disease-Specific Care:** Includes Acute Stroke Ready Hospital, Chronic Kidney Disease, Chronic Obstructive Pulmonary Disease, Comprehensive Stroke Center, Heart Failure, Inpatient Diabetes Care, Lung Volume Reduction Surgery, Primary Stroke Center, Total Hip and Total Knee Replacement, and Ventricular Assist Device Destination Therapy • **Advanced Certification for Palliative Care** • **Behavioral Health Home Certification** (for behavioral health facilities) • **Community-Based Palliative Care Certification** (for home care organizations) • **Comprehensive Cardiac Care Certification** • **Health Care Staffing Services Certification** • **Integrated Care Certification** • **Disease-Specific Care Certification:** Core certification for programs within a medical center or in the community specializing in certain procedures, conditions, and diagnoses • **Medication Compounding Certification** • **Memory Care Certification** (for nursing care centers) • **Patient Blood Management Certification** • **Perinatal Care Certification** • **Post-Acute Care Certification** (for nursing care centers) • **Primary Care Medical Home Certification** (for ambulatory health care, hospitals, and critical access hospitals

measures (*see* Chapter 1). Other resources valued by customers include the Leading Practice Library, and BoosterPaks™. These resources are described in Sidebar 2-1 on page 68.

Conversation Starters
Accreditation as a Proven Approach

- *What types of Joint Commission support resources do we routinely use and in what ways?*
- *Who in our organization should be accessing Joint Commission support resources?*
- *How can we ensure access and appropriate, effective use of these materials?*

Accreditation as a Value Equation

There are financial advantages to accreditation as well. The ACA's VBP program links reimbursement to quality of care. This makes it more important than ever to consider how accreditation by The Joint Commission can support financial health. External research has shown that Joint Commission–accredited hospitals perform better on key financial metrics than hospitals using other accreditors or certification by the Centers for Medicare & Medicaid Services (CMS) alone.[2] Joint Commission–accredited hospitals also have higher net income, higher operating margins, and higher bed occupancy.[2] Studies have also shown that Joint Commission–accredited nursing homes report a more favorable resident safety culture than those without accreditation[3] and a consistent pattern of better performance across a broad range of indicators, including survey deficiencies, quality ratings, and staffing.[4] And research on core measure performance[5] and emergency department effectiveness measures[6] correlates improved quality with Joint Commission hospital accreditation.

Alignment with federal requirements. Joint Commission accreditation is usually used to provide "deemed status" (where relevant) to health care organizations who rely on Medicare and Medicaid reimbursement. This is possible because the requirements for Joint Commission accreditation meet or exceed the standards

SIDEBAR 2-1

Joint Commission Quality and Safety Resources

Resources from The Joint Commission enterprise are invaluable tools in the effort to improve patient safety and provide high-quality care. Information on the following resources and other useful tools can be found through the Joint Commission website at www.jointcommission.org unless otherwise noted:

- ***Core Measure Solution Exchange®:*** A database of success stories from accredited hospitals that have achieved and sustained excellent performance on core measures. Offered only to accredited organizations via *Joint Commission Connect*™ (*see* page 65).
- ***Enterprise Content Library Index:*** A free online resource, updated quarterly, that indexes current content for customers available from The Joint Commission, Joint Commission Resources, Joint Commission International, and the Joint Commission Center for Transforming Healthcare. The Index provides links, organized into topic areas, to hundreds of webpages, articles, books, monographs, videos, webinars, podcasts, FAQs, lessons, and more.
- ***Joint Commission Resources:*** A component of the enterprise that provides print and electronic publications, educational events and courses, consulting services on accreditation and PI, and software that support the mission of quality and safety (*see* www.jcrinc.com).
- ***Leadership Blog:*** A free online blog written by leaders at The Joint Commission that promotes the sharing of knowledge and information to support and inspire health care professionals in their efforts to improve health care for the future.
- ***Leading Practice Library:*** An online library of safety solutions that have been used successfully by health care organizations and reviewed by Joint Commission standards experts. The library is free to Joint Commission–accredited and –certified organizations through the *Joint Commission Connect* extranet. Listings of the resources are also published in the Enterprise Content Library Index.
- ***Oro™ 2.0:*** An online High Reliability Organizational Assessment and resource library to facilitate the discovery of opportunities to improve performance on the high reliability journey—that is, striving for zero patient harm. The assessment guides senior leaders through questions and discussions that identify the organization's strengths and opportunities for improvement. The tool, available to accredited organizations through the Joint Commission Center for Transforming Healthcare, directs the users to appropriate resources (*see* www.centerfortransforminghealthcare.org/oro.aspx.).

- ***Quality and safety portals:*** Dedicated web portals available on the Joint Commission enterprise websites that offer free resources related to quality and safety, including portals on the following topics:
  - Ebola preparedness
  - Emergency management
  - Health equity
  - High reliability
  - Infection prevention and HAIs
  - Pain management
  - Patient safety
  - Physical environment
  - Sentinel events
  - Transitions of care
  - Workplace violence prevention
- ***Physician Leader Monthly:*** A free monthly online newsletter that touches on current issues and topics relevant to physician leaders. Links in the documents lead the reader to more in-depth information.
- ***Quick Safety!:*** Another free monthly online newsletter that outlines an incident, topic, or trend in health care that could compromise patient safety. This newsletter helps Joint Commission–accredited organizations recognize potential safety issues they may encounter.
- ***R^3 Report:*** Requirement, Rationale, Reference: A free online briefing that supports the health care organization's internal communication with its staff about the new requirements and the underlying evidence that is driving the change. *R^3 Reports* are issued when The Joint Commission releases complex new or revised requirements.
- ***Sentinel Event Alert:*** A free online bulletin that identifies a specific type of sentinel event, describes its common causes, and recommends steps to reducing associated risks. These *Alerts* are valuable to organizations in identifying potential areas for improvement (*see* page 94).
- ***Speak Up™ Campaign:*** An award-winning patient safety program that's aimed at encouraging patients to participate in their health care. Materials, most of which are free (including popular animated videos), address such topics as pain, patient advocacy, and preventing medical and medicine errors.
- ***Standards BoosterPak™:*** A document that provides detailed information about a single standard or topic area that's complex and therefore often results in a high volume of inquiries or noncompliance scores. BoosterPaks, available free to accredited organizations through the *Joint Commission Connect* extranet, are designed to give consistency to organizations' understanding of standards interpretation.

continued on page 70

- ***Targeted Solutions Tool® (TST®):*** A step-by-step guide to help health care organizations measure their actual performance, identify barriers to excellent performance, and direct them to implement proven, customized solutions. The TST is offered through the Joint Commission Center for Transforming Healthcare (*see* www.centerfortransforminghealthcare.org/tst.aspx.) and is available for the following four topics:
  - Hand hygiene
  - Hand-off communications
  - Preventing falls
  - Safe surgery
- ***The Joint Commission Perspectives:*** A monthly publication designated as the official publication of The Joint Commission and the primary source for changes to accreditation and certification standards, requirements, and Joint Commission initiatives, including any scoring and decision processes. This periodical is free to accredited organizations through the *Joint Commission Connect* extranet and is also available for purchase from Joint Commission Resources (*see* www.jcrinc.com).

set by CMS. The Joint Commission has deeming authority granted by CMS for hospitals, critical access hospitals, ambulatory surgery centers, advanced diagnostic imaging, home health, hospice, durable medical equipment, and laboratories. By aligning Joint Commission requirements with those of CMS, hospitals and other organizations that choose deemed status can eliminate redundant data collection, reporting efforts, and surveys.

In addition, The Joint Commission's close relationships with federal agencies, such as CMS, the Centers for Disease Control and Prevention, the US Food and Drug Administration, and the Agency for Healthcare Research and Quality, means that The Joint Commission is at the forefront of upcoming legislation and regulations. For example, the Joint Commission's recent development of an antimicrobial stewardship standard for hospitals, critical access hospitals, and nursing care centers supports the National Action Plan for Combating Antibiotic-resistant Bacteria (www.whitehouse.gov/sites/default/files/docs/national_action_plan_for_combating_antibotic-resistant_bacteria.pdf). Accredited organizations can trust that The Joint Commission will be ready to help them adapt and meet new requirements as they emerge.

Call to Action
Accreditation as a Value Equation

It's the responsibility of the board to understand how Joint Commission accreditation and certification enables the health care organization's quality and safety improvement goals. Receiving information about quality and safety indicators at each board meeting is as essential to a board member's fiduciary responsibility as receiving the organization's financial results. It's equally important to be up-to-date on quality and safety requirements from local, state, and federal agencies. Regular review of health care issues, such as those covered in Joint Commission communications and other industry publications, can help you guide your organization in responding to changes—and opportunities—in health care. If your organization has professionals dedicated to regulatory compliance and/or Joint Commission accreditation coordination, they should regularly report to the board on any issues that affect your organization.

Accreditation Requirements

Joint Commission accreditation is based on an organization's compliance with Joint Commission requirements. These requirements comprise a set of standards and National Patient Safety Goals (NPSGs). It's helpful to board members like yourself to know what's meant by the following terms that describe these requirements, as they'll be used frequently in discussions of Joint Commission compliance efforts:

- ***Standard:*** As defined by The Joint Commission, this is a principle of patient safety and quality of care that a well-run organization meets. A standard defines the performance expectations, structures, or processes that must be substantially in place in an organization to enhance the quality of care, treatment, or services.
- ***Element of performance:*** A standard is further broken down into elements of performance (EPs). An EP spells out any specific action(s), process(es), or structure(s) that must be implemented to achieve the goal of a standard. The scoring of EP compliance for a standard determines an organization's overall compliance with that standard.

- **National Patient Safety Goal:** An NPSG describes specific actions that accredited organizations are required to take to ensure patient safety, such as miscommunication among caregivers. A panel of national safety experts has confirmed that taking these simple, proven steps will reduce the frequency of devastating medical errors. (A brief description of the NPSGs for 2016 can be found in Sidebar 2-2 on page 74.)

These requirements represent important protocols, processes, or functions essential to provide safe, high-quality care, including, for example, performance measurement (*see* page 84). The requirements are developed with input from health care professionals, health care organizations, professional associations, subject matter experts, consumers, government agencies, and employers. And they're based on scientific evidence, emerging research, and expert consensus. All requirements are thoroughly evaluated regarding their positive impact on health care, whether they meet or surpass laws and regulations, and if they can be accurately measured by the accreditation survey process (discussed later in this chapter).

Accreditation manuals. The requirements are compiled into comprehensive accreditation manuals specific to each health care program or setting that The Joint Commission accredits and certifies. These manuals include explanations of why each standard and patient safety goal is important, provide a rationale for each, and offer useful information about relevant Joint Commission policies. Electronic editions of the manuals (known as E-dition®) are available free to accredited and certified organizations through the *Joint Commission Connect*™ extranet. Print versions are available for a fee from Joint Commission Resources at www.jcrinc.com.

Accreditation Requirements for the Board

The "Leadership" (LD) standards spell out the responsibilities of an organization's board (using the term *governing body* for the board). The LD standards are designed to help the board, chief executive officer, leaders of the medical staff, and other executives work collaboratively toward quality and safety improvements. The board's responsibilities, per the LD standards, are summarized as follows:

- ***Defining the mission, setting goals, and planning:*** Board members must participate in creating the organization's mission and vision and defining its goals, which are the heart of all strategic and long-term plans. The board must ensure that these values and goals are communicated effectively to everyone in the organization.

- ***Ensuring safety and quality of care:*** The board is ultimately responsible for the organization's provision of safe, high-quality care. Board members must approach all decisions, prioritizing, and resourcing in ways that support improving and sustaining quality and safety. The "Patient Safety Systems" (PS) chapter addresses safety as it relates to leadership, and is discussed in greater detail later in this chapter.
- ***Creating a culture of safety:*** Board members must foster an organizational culture in which honest and open communication is a top priority. The board must not only define behaviors that are acceptable and unacceptable, but model those acceptable behaviors to increase trust and accountability organizationwide. Safety culture was introduced in Chapter 1 and is described later in this chapter in relation to high reliability.
- ***Resolving conflicts:*** The board must establish a conflict resolution system to deal with the inevitable tension among competing priorities and sometimes among individuals. This should include conflicts among board members and medical staff members. Similarly, boards are responsible for managing conflicts of interest by establishing policies to address the identification, disclosure, and resolution.
- ***Assigning responsibilities:*** Boards must identify individuals who'll be responsible for certain tasks within the organization. These tasks include planning, management, and financial and operational responsibilities as well as provision of care, treatment, and services.
- ***Providing resources:*** The board must provide the necessary resources for patient care, focusing on patient safety, staffing, and PI. This includes providing financial support, competent personnel, and other sufficient resources to complete necessary operations as well as quality and safety improvements.
- ***Being accountable:*** The board must assess and improve its own conduct. This means establishing policies and procedures for the board, understanding its role in organizational leadership, and evaluating its ability to carry out its duties.

Other chapters in the accreditation manual reference the LD standards and reinforce the central role that leadership plays. For example, Emergency Management (EM) standards reference the LD standard that requires senior leadership to review annual emergency management planning, and Nursing (NR) standards about nurse executive responsibilities reference LD standards.

SIDEBAR 2-2

National Patient Safety Goals

National Patient Safety Goals (NPSGs) apply to all accreditation programs, so it's important to check the appropriate accreditation manual to ensure compliance. The major NPSGs and the issues they each address are summarized as follows:

- ***Identify patients correctly:*** Safe care is dependent on providing the right care to the right patient. Patients must be identified accurately to make sure they get the right medication and treatment. Multiple pieces of identifying data help ensure that no mistakes are made.
- ***Improve communication among caregivers:*** It's critical that information be provided to the right caregiver in a timely way. For example, test results can indicate a life-threatening situation and must be shared as soon as possible.
- ***Use medicines safely:*** Medication errors can cause serious adverse events. To minimize the risk of these errors, medication must be labeled appropriately and legibly. Also, staff should know what current and new medications a patient is taking, and patients must be given information about all their medications to make sure they know what to take as well as when and how to take it. Extra care is needed for patients who take anticoagulants and insulin.
- ***Use alarms safely:*** Alarm fatigue is a major factor that compromises patient safety. To minimize those risks, an organization should evaluate the alarms on critical medical equipment to ensure that alarms are heard and responded to on time. In some situations, individual alarms may be difficult to detect if there are numerous alarm signals or too many devices with alarms. This may lead to desensitized staff who then miss, ignore, or even disable the alarm signals. Other issues associated with effective alarm system management include default settings that aren't at an actionable level and alarm limits that are too narrow.
- ***Prevent infection:*** Health care–associated infections are widespread yet largely preventable. Proper hand hygiene, as defined by the Centers for Disease Control and Prevention and the World Health Organization, is a simple yet effective way to prevent the spread of infectious particles. In addition, organizations should use proven guidelines to prevent infections caused by multidrug-resistant organisms, central line–associated blood infections, surgical site infections, and indwelling catheter–associated urinary tract infections.
- ***Prevent patient harm from falls:*** Falls are a significant risk in any setting, but in particular for hospitals, nursing care centers, and home care organizations. Patients should be assessed to identify their particular fall risks. The

patient, family or significant others (if applicable), and staff should be trained in fall reduction strategies.

- ***Prevent pressure ulcers:*** Health care–associated pressure ulcers are a significant risk for nursing care center patients. Organizations must identify those patients at risk for pressure ulcers, and take steps to prevent them from occurring, including educating staff on the use of relevant risk assessment tools.
- ***Identify patients at risk for suicide:*** Patient suicide is a risk in any health care environment, but is of particular concern for psychiatric hospitals and any unit that treats patients with emotional or behavioral disorders. Patients should be assessed for risk of suicide during their treatment, and any immediate safety needs should be addressed. At discharge, suicide prevention information should be given to any at-risk patients and/or their family or significant others.
- ***Identify risk of home fires associated with home oxygen therapy:*** Using oxygen at home increases the risk of fires. Before a patient begins oxygen therapy at home, organizations must identify risk factors, such as whether there are smoking materials or open flames present and whether smoke alarms are functioning. Patients, families, significant others, and/or caregivers must be informed of these risks and educated on how to mitigate fire risk.
- ***Prevent mistakes in surgery (Universal Protocol):*** The Universal Protocol applies to all surgical and nonsurgical invasive procedures. It's designed to make sure that the correct procedure is done on the correct patient and at the correct place on the patient's body. This involves conducting a preprocedure verification process, marking the site, and doing a "time-out" before the procedure to conduct a final assessment.

Source: The Joint Commission. 2016 National Patient Safety Goals. Accessed Oct 12, 2016. http://www.jointcommission.org/standards_information/npsgs.aspx.

The Joint Commission Accreditation Process

Accreditation, as noted, isn't a simple evaluation or business transaction. And it's not a one-time event or even a series of events. It's an ongoing process. The accreditation process is usually a three-year cycle that includes an on-site survey, survey follow-up actions and reports, and continuous compliance activities. Figure 2-1 on page 76 presents a graphic summary of accreditation cycle activities, which will be described in this section. (Please refer to "The Accreditation Process" chapter in the appropriate Joint Commission accreditation manual for your organization's program/setting for a more detailed explanation.)

FIGURE 2-1: Key Milestones in the Accreditation Cycle

This time line shows the accreditation process, which is a three-year cycle (except for laboratories, which are on a two-year-cycle). The triennial survey can occur anytime between 18 and 36 months following the previous full, unannounced (if seeking deemed status) survey. Certification cycles, on the other hand, vary. For example, the average cycle for Disease-Specific Care Certification is two years, but the cycle for Primary Care Medical Home Certification and Integrated Care Certification is three years. Check the appropriate certification program for details.

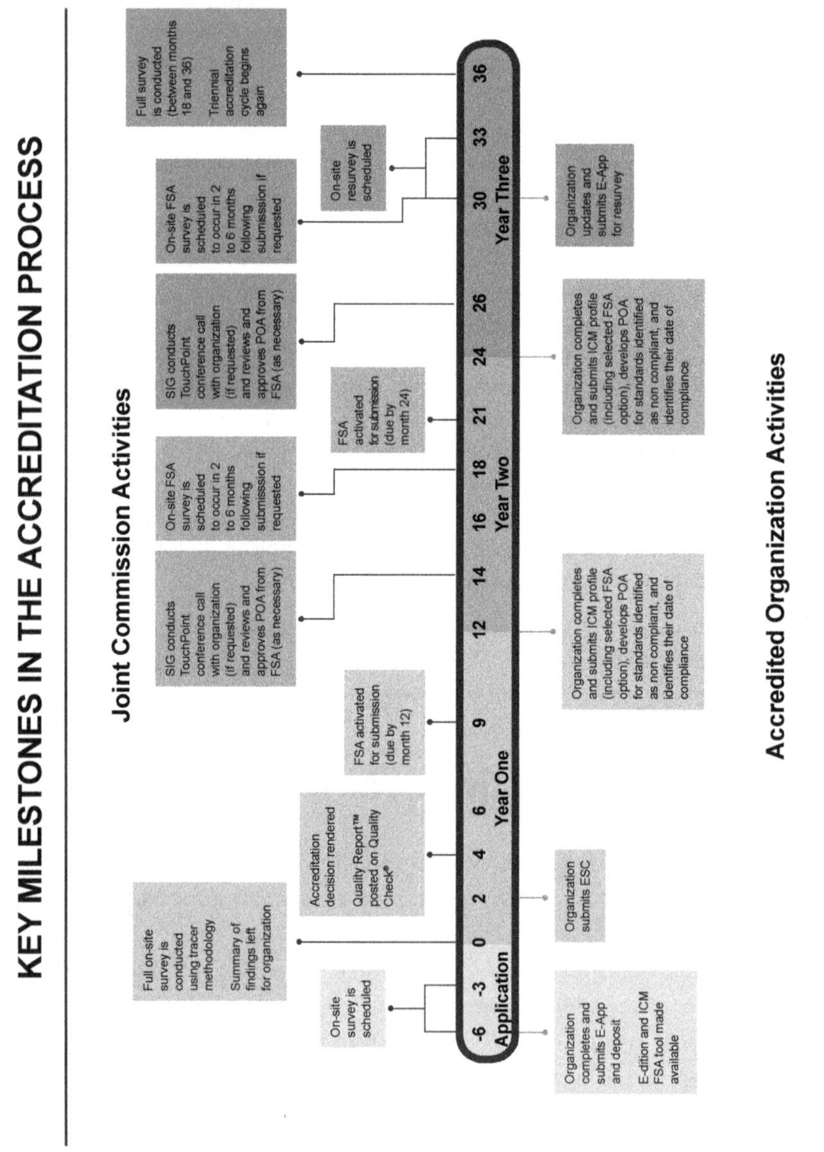

* Activities The Joint Commission completes appear above the time line; activities conducted by the ambulatory care organization appear below the time line.

FSA, Focused Standards Assessment; SIG, Standards Interpretation Group; POA, Plan of Action; E-App, electronic application; ICM, Intracycle Monitoring; ESC, Evidence of Standards Compliance.

The On-Site Survey

Surveying on-site is the primary method The Joint Commission uses to determine an organization's compliance with its standards, which is used to decide its accreditation or certification status (as explained earlier). If a survey is used for deeming purposes, surveyors will assess compliance with the CMS Conditions of Participation (CoPs) or Conditions for Coverage (CfCs) as well as Joint Commission standards and NPSGs.

Before the survey. These accreditation surveys are, with a few exceptions, unannounced. Your organization can have an unannounced survey anytime between 18 and 36 months after its previous full unannounced survey; the length of the survey will vary based on the size of your organization and the complexity of its care and services.

Being prepared for an unannounced survey is part of being successful. This means doing a certain amount of work before the survey, such as having a plan for what to do when the surveyors show up, ensuring that all documentation is up to date and easily accessible, and educating everyone on what happens during and after a survey. A survey readiness committee is a good idea, if your organization doesn't already have one.

During the survey. An accreditation survey may vary from one to five days depending on your organization's size and scope of services and whether it's your first survey or not. The survey focuses on patient-centered processes and organization functions that support quality and safety. Joint Commission surveyors (there may be one or several) assess an organization's compliance by doing the following:

- Following (tracing) the care delivered to patients and the information transfer among staff and across settings/sites of care (*see* page 79)
- Reviewing verbal and written information provided by the organization
- Observing processes and talking with leaders, staff members, and patients
- Reviewing documents provided by the organization

For the accreditation survey to be effective, your organization must participate in good faith. This means that all staff (including medical staff) must cooperate completely with the Joint Commission surveyor(s). As leaders, you should be sure that the culture of safety carries over into the survey process. Open communication is vital. Staff, patients, and families and/or significant others should feel comfortable sharing information and concerns with the surveyor(s).

During the leadership session (part of the survey), surveyors engage leadership in a discussion of the organization's governance, management, information systems, infrastructure, and key patient care and support processes, as they relate to quality indicators, patient safety, a culture of safety, and Robust Process Improvement® (RPI®) (*see* page 102).

Then, while still on site, the surveyor(s) will prepare, present, and leave a preliminary Summary of Survey Findings Report on the findings, discussing areas of concern with senior leaders and the board, if available. This report details observations the surveyors made about the organization's compliance with Joint Commission standards, NPSGs, and the CMS CoPs (if it's a deeming survey). The findings identify the specific areas where your organization might have increased risks related to quality and safety.

After the survey. For every standard, NPSG, and CMS CoP (if it's a deeming survey) found noncompliant during the survey, your organization will receive a Requirement for Improvement (RFI). Organizations must respond to every RFI by submitting an Evidence of Standards Compliance (ESC) report. There are two types of ESC, as follows:

- ***Corrective ESC:*** This details what actions were taken to bring the organization into compliance. A corrective ESC must address compliance at the EP level for all applicable corrections. The time line for submitting a corrective ESC is 60 days.
- ***Clarifying ESC:*** If the organization believes it was in compliance at the time of survey, it may submit this type of ESC, which includes an explanation and proof of compliance, such as results of an audit. The clarifying ESC must be submitted within 10 business days following the posting of the organization's report on the extranet.

The Accreditation Decision

Two weeks to two months after the survey (depending on required follow-up activity), The Joint Commission renders its accreditation decision. The decision is awarded for three years (except for laboratory accreditation, which is awarded for two years).

Possible outcomes. The outcomes differ depending on whether the survey is an initial survey or a renewal, as described:

- ***Initial survey:*** The decision process for any organization undergoing an initial Joint Commission survey may result in either Accredited or Denial of

Call to Action
The On-Site Survey

Boards can help their organizations improve throughout the survey process. Before the survey, boards can incentivize leaders to declare and implement initiatives to reduce harm and remind leaders that the purpose of the evaluation process is to identify risks so they can be addressed before harm occurs. During the survey, board members should participate in the leadership session. After the survey, boards should request updates on improvements made as a result of survey results. Board members may wish to participate in safety rounds or daily huddles to remain informed and further demonstrate their commitment to safety.

Accreditation outcomes. The organization must demonstrate the capability to meet Joint Commission standards before it can be rendered an Accredited decision.

- ***Renewal:*** Organizations seeking to renew their accreditation are subject to the full range of decisions, which include Denial of Accreditation, Preliminary Denial of Accreditation, Contingent Accreditation, Accreditation with Follow-up Survey, Preliminary Accreditation, and Accredited.

Tracer Methodology

Tracers are a central component of an accreditation survey. This activity assesses the actual experience of patients as they receive care and move through the organization, or traces key processes of care, information transfer, and other processes and structures (such as those related to the physical environment of care). Mock tracers that simulate actual survey tracers can be performed by the organization itself to assess its own performance, identify areas for improvement, or prepare for survey. Many organizations have a mock tracer program as part of their survey readiness and PI efforts.

There are three general types of tracers: individual, program-specific, and system tracers.

Individual tracers. Individual tracers are designed to follow a patient through his or her care experience. During a survey, the surveyor(s) tries to select patients with experiences that will give the best representation of the organization. Surveyors often choose patients who have had care that crosses programs/settings, such as a nursing care center resident who is admitted to the hospital and then is transferred to a rehabilitation facility. Those whose care brings them into contact with key risk areas, such as infection control or medication management, are also frequently selected patients to trace. The idea is to have individual tracers that reflect the patient experience in the organization's systems, both as stand-alone components and as they work together across the continuum of care.

Program-specific tracers. Program-specific tracers aim to identify safety concerns within different levels and types of care. They focus on important issues relevant to the organization, such as clinical services offered and high-risk or high-volume patient populations. Not all surveys will include a program-specific tracer. One example of a program-specific tracer for hospitals is laboratory integration. This tracer evaluates how the laboratory interacts with the various areas of the hospital, such as specimen collection, handling, and test result reporting.

System tracers. System tracers focus on a specific system or process across the entire organization. The surveyor(s) will try to use specific patients' experiences whenever possible. The following topics may be covered by a system tracer during survey:

- ***Data management:*** How the organization collects, analyzes, interprets, and uses data to improve care and safety; performed on every survey
- ***Infection control:*** How the organization complies with infection prevention and control standards
- ***Medication management:*** How the organization manages medication, from procurement to administration to monitoring for effect on patients, focusing on potential risk points

Other tracers. Which types of tracers are used depends on what kind of organization is being surveyed and what the surveyor(s) observes. The following are some other common types of tracers:

- ***Environment of care tracer*:** A tracer similar to a system tracer that focuses on the physical environment of a health care organization
- **Life Safety Code®*** ***assessment:*** A tracer, conducted by *Life Safety Code* surveyors, that involves a document review of pertinent policies, procedures, and testing and maintenance activities related to life (fire) safety as well as a building tour

* *Life Safety Code®* is a registered trademark of the National Fire Protection Association, Quincy, MA.

Patient flow tracers for leaders. When conducting any kind of tracer, the surveyor(s) will interview staff who are involved with providing care or who participate in the process being assessed. If a surveyor sees something that triggers the need for a patient flow tracer, leaders will be involved because this topic is the responsibility of leadership under Joint Commission LD standards. A patient flow tracer looks at how patients move through an organization. This is an important concern because poor patient flow can cause treatment delays, medical errors, or unsafe practices. Patient flow problems can occur anywhere in an organization, although the emergency departments of hospitals are frequent focus areas.

Conversation Starters
Tracer Methodology

- *Does our organization have a mock tracer program, and if so, how does it operate?*
- *What types of system- and program-specific tracers are typically part of our surveys?*
- *When was the last time we had a patient flow tracer, and what did it reveal?*

Risk Classification and the SAFER™ Matrix

Throughout the tracers that occur during survey, Joint Commission surveyors will identify and communicate risk levels associated with deficiencies through a transformative approach known as the Survey Analysis for Evaluating Risk (SAFER). This approach provides organizations with additional information related to the risk level of deficiencies to help prioritize and focus corrective actions. The SAFER Matrix (*see* Figure 2-2, page 82) is a graphic approach for communicating those risk levels associated with standards noncompliance cited during surveys.

Benefits of SAFER: This approach includes the following benefits:

- Helps leaders more easily identify higher risk RFIs
- Identifies the potential for widespread quality initiatives
- Better organizes survey findings by level of potential patient impact
- Provides one comprehensive visual representation of survey findings

FIGURE 2-2: The SAFER™ Matrix

The Survey Analysis for Evaluating Risk (SAFER) approach and matrix provides accredited organizations the information needed to prioritize resources and focus corrective actions where they're needed most. Joint Commission surveyors will plot each Requirement for Improvement (RFI) on the SAFER matrix according to the likelihood the RFI could cause harm and the scope at which the RFI was observed. As risk level of the RFI increases, the placement of the standard and element of performance (EP) will move from bottom left corner (lowest risk) to the upper right corner (highest risk).

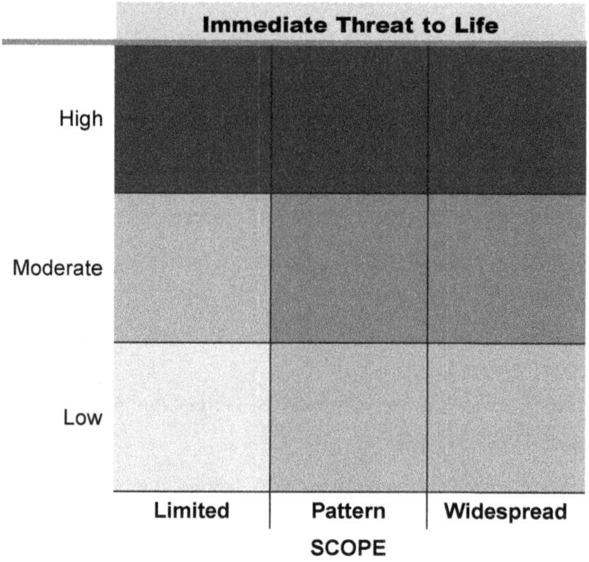

Continuous Compliance

Most Joint Commission surveys are once every three years, but that doesn't mean that safety and quality of care are only important once every three years. It's expected that your organization be in continuous compliance with all applicable standards and EPs at all times. The Joint Commission may request compliance information between surveys, and may schedule additional surveys at any time in response to concerns about patient safety. For example, patient safety specialists from the Joint Commission Office of Quality and Patient Safety may conduct an off-cycle on-site review in response to a complaint about an organization made to The Joint Commission (*see* page 94).

Currently, The Joint Commission requires an acknowledgement of a self-assessment activity at the 12th and 24th month for most programs, and at the 12th month for the lab program. The Joint Commission offers tools and support to help complete this self-assessment and maintain continuous compliance. The primary method provided is the Intracycle Monitoring (ICM) Profile, which is available through the *Joint Commission Connect* extranet site.

Intracycle Monitoring Profile. The ICM Profile is an interactive, user-friendly workspace that helps organizations maintain their compliance on an ongoing basis. The ICM Profile guides an organization through self-assessment, design of PI activities, and monitoring of results by providing the following:

- ***Activity tracking:*** Tracking of past and current survey follow-up activities, such as the Accreditation Survey Findings Report
- ***Resource links:*** Links to relevant Joint Commission tools, materials from CMS, newsletters, publications, and other resources
- ***Standards guidance:*** Opportunity to seek guidance from the Standards Interpretation Group about specific concerns

Focused Standards Assessment. The central component of the ICM Profile is the Focused Standards Assessment (FSA) tool, which helps organizations incorporate standards compliance into everyday operations. While the FSA will list all the standards that are applicable to an organization, it highlights those that fall into identified risk areas, using the special R icon. This icon is used to mark standards that are one or more of the following:

- National Patient Safety Goals
- Joint Commission–identified risk areas
- RFIs identified during the current accreditation cycle survey events

Onsite ICM. In addition to the FSA tool, organizations have these two ICM assessment options:

- ***An on-site educational survey with documented findings:*** Following the on-site survey, an organization has 30 days to develop and submit plans of action for any findings documented by the surveyor.
- ***An on-site educational survey that does not include documented findings:*** Following an oral exit briefing by the surveyor, the assessment concludes.

Quality Reports® and Quality Check®

After a survey has been conducted and an accreditation decision has been reached, The Joint Commission provides organizations with a Quality Report, which serves as a report of reference for compliance efforts. It also serves as a report of reference for the public. Information from these reports is posted on The Joint Commission's Quality Check website (www.qualitycheck.org). Quality Check acts as a directory for the more than 21,000 Joint Commission–accredited and –certified organizations and programs in the United States. It includes multiple search options, such as name of the organization, geographic location, accreditation and certification program(s), and type(s) of services provided.

On the Quality Check website, the public can view and download a Quality Report for each Joint Commission–accredited and –certified organization. This information includes the following about the organization:

- Accreditation and certification status
- Standards compliance problem areas (for organizations with a status other than Accredited, Accredited with Follow-Up Survey, or Certified)
- Locations and services offered
- National Patient Safety Goals compliance
- Hospital performance measurement set results (*see* page 86)

An organization may include a commentary (up to two pages) to accompany its Quality Report; this is completely voluntary.

The Joint Commission and Measurement

Compliance issues highlighted in the report from an accreditation survey will almost certainly be incorporated into PI efforts. The results are, in fact, a type of performance measurement data, the foundation of PI work. Making sure you have good measures, ones that hold you accountable for actual improvement in quality and safety, is critical.

Accountability Measures

The Joint Commission has designated some of its performance measures as "accountability measures" as an added method of promoting high-quality care and improved patient outcomes. Accountability measures produce the greatest positive impact on patient outcomes as demonstrated by hospitals and critical access hospitals.

Criteria for accountability measures: All accountability measures meet the following four criteria:

- ***Accuracy:*** The measure accurately assesses whether or not the care process has actually been provided.

- ***Adverse effects:*** Implementing the measure has little or no chance of inducing unintended adverse consequences.
- ***Proximity:*** Performing the care process is closely connected to the outcome.
- ***Research:*** Strong scientific evidence demonstrates that performing the evidence-based care process improves health outcomes.

Not all standardized measures meet these criteria. However, these measures still have value as guidelines for providing appropriate patient care. The Joint Commission works to eliminate measures that don't work well in representing the actual care delivered. It has integrated accountability measures, along with other standardized measures, into the information reported on the Quality Check website and includes accountability measures in the ORYX initiative (*see* below). The Joint Commission reports all standardized measures data received with the exception of hospital outpatient measures and those measures that it deems "risk-adjusted" measures. The only condition for measures to be reported on Quality Check is that the measure be endorsed by the National Quality Forum (*see* Chapter 1).

Conversation Starters
Accountability Measures

- *What type of standardized measures does our organization use in performance measurement?*
- *Do our measures meet the criteria of the accountability measures?*
- *If not, are we actively moving toward use of those criteria?*

The ORYX® Initiative

One of the primary ways that performance measurement data are integrated into the accreditation process is through the ORYX initiative. As introduced in Chapter 1, ORYX is an overarching term for The Joint Commission's performance measure reporting requirement for hospitals. It necessitates the reporting of data on measures, not all of which are accountability measures (*see* page 86 for ORYX requirements).

ORYX standardized performance measures sets. ORYX relies on data derived from standardized measures with precisely defined data elements, calculation algorithms, and consistent data collection protocols that focus on specific conditions and patient populations. These measures are grouped into sets. Current measure sets cover the following:

- Emergency department
- Hospital-based inpatient psychiatric services
- Hospital outpatient department
- Immunization
- Perinatal care
- Stroke
- Substance use
- Tobacco treatment
- Venous thromboembolism

ORYX requirements. Participation in ORYX and the use of its measures is mandatory for Joint Commission–accredited hospitals and critical access hospitals. The requirements are as follows:

- ***Six-set minimum:*** Most Joint Commission–accredited hospitals must collect and transmit data to The Joint Commission on a minimum of six sets of the measures. Selection of measure sets is at the discretion of the hospital and will vary from one organization to another, depending on the services provided and patient populations served. Exceptions are as follows:
  - Small hospitals (fewer than 10 inpatients daily census) need to collect data internally, but don't need to transmit that data to The Joint Commission.
  - Critical access hospitals need only collect internal data on four sets and aren't required to transmit the data to The Joint Commission.
  - Joint Commission–accredited freestanding psychiatric hospitals are only required to collect and transmit the hospital-based inpatient psychiatric services measure set.
  - All hospitals that provide obstetrical services and have at least 300 live births per year are required to collect data on the perinatal care measure set and transmit that along with the other selected sets to The Joint Commission.
- ***Quarterly submission via vendors:*** Data for all applicable measures in each set selected must be submitted through performance measurement system vendors that have been evaluated and listed by The Joint Commission. Vendors submit monthly de-identified patient-level data to The Joint Commission on a quarterly basis. Those data are then used to generate the ORYX Performance Measure Report.

ORYX Performance Measure Report. Following a hospital's required quarterly submission of ORYX data, The Joint Commission processes those data through the measure algorithms. It then generates an ORYX Performance Measure Report and posts it on each hospital's secure *Joint Commission Connect* extranet site.

The quarterly report provides the hospital with a summary analysis of its performance at the measure set level and for each individual measure. Through the use of control charts and "target" charts created for each measure, the hospital gets information on the stability over time of the process addressed by each measure. The reports also analyze the hospital's predicted range of performance against a measure target range that's based on the national rate of performance on each core measure. Board members often receive these summary reports or highlights from the hospital administration as part of regular PI data reports, so look for it and examine it carefully.

Survey assessment of ORYX data. At the time of survey, Joint Commission surveyors also look carefully at the ORYX data and assess the following in relation to them:

- The hospital's integration and use of ORYX data into internal PI activities
- The hospital's data collection processes (such as data accuracy, reliability, and security)
- The hospital's data analysis methodologies and related training
- The dissemination of findings

When poor performance against the national target for a specific measure for two of the most recent four quarters is identified, the hospital will be expected to provide the surveyor with evidence of a credible analysis of its outlier status on the measure.

eCQMs as ORYX options. Collecting, analyzing, and reporting on performance measurement data is a big job, but it's becoming easier and more efficient with advances in technology. Traditionally, performance measurement data were collected from paper records and entered electronically to be transmitted by the vendor. Recent health care reforms have pushed for the adoption of electronic health records (EHRs), which has in turn created the opportunity to draw performance measurement data directly from the EHRs. Measures that can be pulled directly from the EHR are called electronic clinical quality measures (eCQMs).

The Joint Commission has responded to this development by creating additional options for ORYX reporting requirements that allow organizations to use a qualifying Joint Commission–listed vendor for the capture and reporting of eCQM data. Not all vendors are currently able to process eCQMs, so not all vendors will qualify. Organizations should therefore evaluate their existing systems and vendor relationships when making decisions regarding their ORYX reporting options.

Pioneers in Quality. To help organizations transition from current measures to eCQMs, The Joint Commission created the Pioneers in Quality program. This effort is designed to provide information and support through a resource portal, educational webinars, peer-to-peer solution exchange, recognition categories, and more. For details on the Pioneers in Quality program, or to access its resources, visit www.jointcommission.org/topics/pioneers_in_quality.aspx.

Library of Other Measures

In addition to the ORYX measures, The Joint Commission maintains a library of PI measures that are reliable and fully tested to improve safety and quality of care. The library includes measures that don't meet the stringent requirements of accountability measures as well as other measures recently developed or specified by The Joint Commission. The latter group includes measures such as those that address intensive care units, nursing-sensitive care, and patient blood management. In the future, the library will include externally developed measures that The Joint Commission has evaluated and determined meet rigorous criteria. More information on these additional measures can be found on the Joint Commission website: www.jointcommission.org/library_of_other_measures.aspx.

Alignment with CMS Measures

Since 2004 The Joint Commission and CMS have been working together to align performance measures common to both organizations. These standardized common measures are called National Hospital Inpatient Quality Measures, and they're integral to safety and quality improvement. Measure alignment benefits hospitals by making it easier and less costly to collect and report data, because the same data set can be used to satisfy both CMS and Joint Commission requirements. All of the National Hospital Inpatient Quality Measures common to The Joint Commission and CMS are endorsed by the National Quality Forum (*see* Chapter 1). Detailed information on standardized measures can be found on the Joint Commission website at www.jointcommission.org/performance_measurement.aspx.

Call to Action
The Joint Commission and Measurement

The performance measurement arena is rapidly changing, with new measures and metrics emerging all the time. Some of these performance measures lack adequate validity and reliability; others are duplicative. You and the other board members need to understand which measures are being used in your organization—particularly which of those are connected to reimbursement and payer requirements as well as which are essential for Joint Commission accreditation and quality/safety improvement efforts. If you don't have this information currently, ask for it.

The Joint Commission and Patient Safety

The overall goal of accreditation and performance measurement is to reduce the risks to patients and ensure that they receive safe, high-quality care. Thus, The Joint Commission has built quality and safety into all aspects of its accreditation process to help organizations incorporate quality and safety into all their improvement efforts. Quality and safety are, after all, inextricably linked: Safety is expected in high-quality health care processes and results. That simple but profoundly important relationship is highlighted in the opening to a chapter in the accreditation manuals that's dedicated to the topic of patient safety systems.

"Patient Safety Systems" (PS) chapter. This chapter of the accreditation manual doesn't contain new requirements; what it does is gather and list all existing standards related to quality and safety from other chapters into one place. It helps organizational leaders understand how Joint Commission standards support quality and safety and stresses the importance and structure of an integrated patient safety system. To that end, it includes guidance on the following topics, which are described in this section:

- ***Learning from patient safety events:*** Becoming a learning organization, where patient safety events are seen as opportunities to learn and improve
- ***Leadership in patient safety:*** Strengthening the role of leadership in patient safety, including the fostering of a safety culture

- ***Reporting and responding to patient safety events:*** Using event reporting systems, appropriate responses, and analysis of events to ensure safety
- ***Risk management to prevent patient safety events:*** Reducing risk of harm through proactive risk assessments
- ***The patient's role in patient safety:*** Encouraging patients' participation in their own care

Learning from Patient Safety Events

In the delivery of everyday health care, things can go wrong that put patients at increased risk of cause or harm. These are patient safety events. A patient safety event is any event, incident, or condition that could have resulted, or did result, in harm to a patient (including "errors"). Patient safety events are broken down into several categories that include the following, as The Joint Commission defines them:

- ***Adverse event:*** A patient safety event that results in harm to a patient
- ***Sentinel event:*** A type of adverse event in which the patient suffers death, permanent harm, or severe temporary harm that is not primarily related to the natural course of the patient's illness or an underlying condition; the term *sentinel event* is used because it signals the need for immediate investigation and response.
- ***Close call (sometimes called "near miss," "no harm," or "good catch"):*** A patient safety event that did not cause harm as defined by the term *sentinel event*
- ***Hazardous condition (sometimes called "unsafe condition"):*** A circumstance (unrelated to the patient's disease process or condition) that increases the probability of an adverse event

The response to patient safety events should involve a "report to learn" approach. In this approach, all patient safety events should be considered learning opportunities, regardless of whether a patient was harmed. Numerous organizations now have daily "safety huddles" to discuss both potential and actual patient safety events, with a goal to prevent future occurrences. Some health systems track the number of days since the last patient safety event and report this information on their internal and/or external websites. Analyzing these events and identifying their underlying causes is valuable to PI efforts.

Conversation Starters
Learning from Patient Safety Events

- *How does the board provide oversight of patient safety events?*
- *Do board members participate in safety rounds?*
- *Does the board see data on health care–acquired conditions?*

Leadership in Patient Safety

Leaders in learning organizations adopt a transparent, nonpunitive approach to reporting so that the organization can collectively learn from patient safety events. That requires a strong safety culture, as introduced in Chapter 1. The safety culture must ensure safety for patients and staff during clinical and nonclinical activities and safety for staff in reporting errors and sharing information related to patient safety. The basic concept: You can't keep people safe unless everyone feels safe to report problems that threaten safety.

Leaders support the safety culture by ensuring that everyone in the whole organization, at all levels, follows a professional code of conduct that spells out acceptable behaviors and those that undermine a culture of safety. In fact, developing this code is an LD standards requirement.

Behaviors that undermine a culture of safety. Behaviors such as intimidation or disrespect must be clearly defined in the code of conduct and appropriately addressed if they occur. These behaviors might include the following:

- Inappropriate words, such as profanity, insults, intimidation, or humiliating or abusive language
- Shaming others for negative outcomes
- Unjustified negative comments or complaints
- Preventing others from providing high-quality care by refusing to comply with known and accepted practice standards
- Not cooperating with others
- Creating unreasonable barriers to communication, including requests for help
- Not returning pages or calls promptly

Behaviors that promote a culture of safety. Leaders, including board members, need to be the greatest proponents for this type of culture, working to build collaborative, nonconfrontational relationships between managers and all levels of staff. They must lead by example, modeling the type of safety- and patient-oriented behavior that's necessary for an effective safety culture. Ways leaders can do this include the following:

- Promoting learning
- Motivating staff
- Providing a transparent environment where information flows freely
- Modeling professional behavior
- Addressing behaviors that might interfere with safety
- Providing resources and training about improvement initiatives

These actions are particularly important when managing change or implementing process improvements (*see* page 119). Change is always challenging, but leadership involvement and role modeling can tip the scales toward success.

Reporting and Responding to Patient Safety Events

As indicated, improving patient safety—and preventing patient safety events—depends in part on staff reports of patient safety events. Leadership—including the board—should be notified of all adverse events through a robust, standardized reporting system and should ensure that the ensuing investigations and corrective actions follow the organization's process for responding to patient safety events. The type of response often depends on the type of patient safety event reported, but there are some basic elements to these responses.

Analysis and action. When a patient safety event is reported, the health care organization needs to determine soon afterward what went wrong. This is done through a comprehensive systematic analysis. While there are several forms this analysis might take, the most common is a root cause analysis (introduced in Chapter 1). This process involves several steps, as follows:

- Identify exactly what occurred.
- Determine what immediate events or factors contributed to the event.
- Identify the underlying causes of the contributing factors, at the most basic level.

When the underlying causes are identified, then an action plan can be developed to reduce the risk of similar events. The plan must describe the following:

- What action will be taken
- Who will be responsible for implementing the action

- Time line and deadlines
- Strategies for evaluating effectiveness and sustaining change

Sentinel Event Policy. A comprehensive systematic analysis is only one part of the response for any sentinel event that occurs. All sentinel events must be reviewed by the organization and are subject to review by The Joint Commission.

Per the Joint Commission Sentinel Event Policy, the organization must respond to a sentinel event with the following:

- Stabilization of the patient or injured person(s)
- Notification of and support for family as well as involved staff
- Notification of leadership
- Immediate investigation
- Comprehensive systematic analysis
- Corrective action plans with time lines
- Systemic improvements

The Joint Commission's Sentinel Event Policy is designed to help organizations that experience serious adverse events to improve safety. The policy encourages voluntary reporting of sentinel events to The Joint Commission and requires that a comprehensive systematic analysis (most commonly a root cause analysis) be conducted.

Benefits of reporting sentinel events. An organization can benefit from voluntarily reporting sentinel events in the following ways:

- ***Support:*** The organization receives support from The Joint Commission during the review of a sentinel event.
- ***Expertise:*** The organization learns from the event by collaborating with Joint Commission patient safety experts.
- ***Transparency:*** The reporting of the event raises the level of transparency at the organization, which promotes a safety culture.
- ***Commitment:*** The reporting of the event conveys the organization's commitment to preventing future patient safety events.

In addition, reporting events contributes de-identified "lessons learned" to The Joint Commission's Sentinel Event Database. This knowledge can help other organizations reduce their own risks, improving safety on a much broader scale. Information in the "Sentinel Events" chapter of the manuals provides guidance on addressing such events.

Sentinel Event Alerts. The Joint Commission periodically publishes *Sentinel Event Alerts* to raise the awareness of changes or developments that affect sentinel events and how they can be prevented. The issues covered in the newsletter are prompted by results from the database of reported incidents, and the recommendations for reducing risks are developed from the experiences of actual organizations and from the advice of experts in the field. *Sentinel Event Alerts* can be found online at www.jointcommission.org/sentinel_event.aspx. They're among the many other patient safety-related resources The Joint Commission enterprise offers. *See* Sidebar 2-1 (page 68) for a description of the key resources available to accredited hospitals.

Conversation Starters

Reporting and Responding to Patient Safety Events

- *What should the board know about sentinel events?*
- *Who gets debriefed on sentinel events?*
- *Are we focusing on taking corrective actions?*
- *Are our corrective actions sustainable?*
- *Do we get routine reports about the impact of the corrective actions?*

Office of Quality and Patient Safety. The Joint Commission's mission to oversee patient safety and quality of care in its accredited organizations relies on sharing information from a variety of sources—including reports of sentinel events. Proactive outreach by organizations about areas of concern in their own organizations is increasing with an eye toward transparency. Common concerns or complaints deal with issues such as patient rights, quality of care, safety, staffing, and medication use. Anyone with a concern or complaint about safety or quality of care should first notify the organization's leaders; however, if the issue remains unresolved, it can be reported to the Joint Commission Office of Quality and Patient Safety by any of the following means:

Online: https://apps.jointcommission.org/QMSInternet/IncidentEntry.aspx
E-mail: patientsafetyreport@jointcommission.org
Fax: 630-792-5636

Mail: The Joint Commission, One Renaissance Boulevard, Oakbrook Terrace, IL 60181

A complaint should include the name and address of the organization and a description of the concern. If follow-up contact is desired, the complainant should include his or her name and address and/or e-mail address. Confidentiality of this information is strictly maintained. More information on reporting concerns and complaints can be found at this webpage: www.jointcommission.org/report_a_complaint.aspx.

Risk Management to Prevent Patient Safety Events

A strong safety culture, with leadership as a core component, and a willingness to report patient safety events and learn from them are vital to building a patient safety system. So is risk management. The Joint Commission standards require accredited organizations to manage risks to make care as safe as possible. Risk management is essentially comprised of the following steps:

Step 1. Identification of the risk
Step 2. Risk analysis and investigation
Step 3. Selection of the best risk management strategy
Step 4. Implementation of the chosen strategy
Step 5. Monitoring the results and making needed modifications

Risk management can take two forms:

- ***Reactive:*** Taking action and making changes in response to a patient safety event
- ***Proactive:*** Identifying risks via risk assessment, and making changes to correct them before those risks cause a patient safety event

Of course, it's always better to prevent harm altogether, which is why the proactive approach is important and why a safety culture that encourages reporting risks is necessary. Proactive risk management is particularly critical in high-risk areas, so The Joint Commission requires organizations to perform periodic proactive risk assessments in such areas.

Essential components of a proactive risk assessment. Risk assessments provide organizations with the opportunity to prevent harm from identified risks. These risks may be unsafe conditions, processes, and/or systems. All proactive risk assessments, however, should include an analysis of any relevant processes or systems as well as the following conditions that may affect or be affected by processes and/or systems:

- ***Preconditions:*** These may include, for example, clutter in a corridor or inadequate staffing.
- ***Supervisory issues:*** Examples of these include failure to address a known problem or authorization of activities known to be risky.
- ***Organizational influences:*** These may be inadequate policies and training, lack of resources to perform processes safely, or even lack of resources to do risk assessments properly.

Common proactive risk assessment tools. Many proactive risk assessment tools are available for your organization to try. The most common are the following:

- ***Failure mode and effects analysis (FMEA):*** This method asks "what if?" to explore what might happen if a particular failure occurs. (*See* Chapter 1 for more about how this compares to a root cause analysis.)
- ***Cause-and-effect diagram:*** Also called a fishbone or Ishikawa diagram, this visual system is used to identify all possible causes of issues that might arise from a particular process or system as well as identify relationships for potential process and/or system improvements.
- ***Potential problem analysis (PPA):*** This is a systematic method to determine what could go wrong if a proposed plan is implemented.
- ***Process decision program chart (PDPC):*** This is a tool used to identify an implementation plan's errors while it's still being created.

Conversation Starters
Risk Management to Prevent Patient Safety Events

- *What is our approach to risk assessment?*
- *What risk assessment tools do we use regularly?*
- *What types of supervisory issues are we seeing that contribute to risks?*
- *What about organizational issues?*

The Patient's Role in Patient Safety

As noted in Chapter 1, patients (and their families and/or significant others) are becoming more involved in their care—a practice that benefits the patients and the health care organization. The patient-centered approach to care supports patient safety in various ways, such as encouraging patients to speak up when they have questions, inviting them to be part of their own care plan team, and helping them to leverage health care information technologies. Patients can also be engaged by making them aware of their rights and responsibilities, which is a Joint Commission requirement.

Principles for patient-centered care. Board members and other leaders need to make patient-centered care a top priority. The "Patient Safety Systems" chapter cites the following principles that can be adopted to guide this approach:

- Patient safety guides all decision making.
- Patients and families (and/or significant others) are partners at every level of care.
- Patient- and family-centered care is verifiable, rewarded, and celebrated.
- Practitioners responsible for the patient's care disclose to the patient and family (and/or significant others) any unanticipated outcomes of care, treatment, and services.
- Physicians disclose harm, express sympathy, and apologize, as appropriate.
- Staffing levels are sufficient, and staff have the necessary tools and skills.
- The hospital has a focus on measurement, learning, and improvement.
- Staff and practitioners are fully engaged in patient- and family-centered care as demonstrated by their skills, knowledge, and competence in compassionate communication.

No matter which principles are applied or which tools and approaches are used, the structure and processes of an integrated patient safety system should be designed to catch weaknesses before they can cause harm, which must be the goal of every health care organization. In recent years, the stated goal of "zero patient harm" has been ushered in via a concept known as "high reliability."

The Joint Commission and High Reliability

The concept of high reliability has traditionally been applied to industries such as commercial aviation and nuclear power. It's only in recent years that it has been applied to health care. The Joint Commission Center for Transforming Healthcare (the Center), for example, has adopted high reliability principles to help transform health care, and it offers guidance to organizations that want to do the same.

High Reliability Principles

Five principles of high reliability effectively summarize the successful practices of high reliability organizations (HROs). These principles are as follows[6]:

- ***Preoccupation with failure:*** Remaining always alert to even the smallest threats to safety, and never becoming satisfied with or complacent about current safety levels
- ***Reluctance to simplify:*** Resisting the temptation to simplify observations and experiences, by understanding that threats to safety can be complex, and also being able to discern the subtle differences among threats
- ***Sensitivity to operations:*** Recognizing that the earliest indicators of threats often occur with small changes in operations, and that those familiar with such processes are most likely to notice such unsafe situations, so they must feel not only free to voice their concerns but obligated to do so
- ***Commitment to resilience:*** Accepting that errors will occur and safety will be threatened, but focusing on identifying errors early and containing them quickly before they can develop into major problems
- ***Deference to expertise:*** Adhering to a mechanism that allows authority for dealing with an issue be given to the person who has the most experience with the issue rather than the person who has the most seniority

Currently, it's not standard practice for health care organizations to use these principles. In fact, most organizations seem to operate without regard to high reliability.[6] Instead of being preoccupied with (or intolerant of) failure, health care organizations have low expectations for safety, accepting failure as routine and inevitable.[6] Poor communication and intimidation among care providers is common, despite standards requiring a culture of safety, and can severely compromise safety. A health care organization's authority structures are often dominated by bureaucratic hierarchy, such as senior physicians dismissing their junior colleagues or pharmacists struggling to be heard in conversations about medication errors.

Framework of Changes for the Journey to High Reliability

The kinds of sweeping changes that need to happen to create HROs in health care cannot, and should not, happen all at once. Rather, organizations should enact a series of incremental changes, working within a framework, to meet defined milestones along the journey to high reliability. The framework for the journey to high reliability championed by The Joint Commission, and promoted by its Center

Conversation Starters
High Reliability Principles

- *Does our organization utilize any of these principles?*
- *Can or should our organization utilize any of these principles?*
- *What barriers do we face in utilizing these principles?*
- *What kind of support—internal and external—might we need to utilize them?*

for Transforming Healthcare, targets the following three major areas of necessary change, each of which will be addressed below:

- Leadership
- Safety culture
- Robust Process Improvement

Each area of change includes specific components (14 components in all). Progress within each component is defined for four "stages of maturity": beginning, developing, advancing, and approaching. Organizations can assess their current stage for each component using the Oro™ 2.0 High Reliability Organizational Assessment, which is available through the Center to all Joint Commission–accredited hospitals and critical access hospitals on *Joint Commission Connect*, the customer extranet (*see* Sidebar 2-1 on page 68) or via the Center's website: http://www.centerfortransforminghealthcare.org/oro.aspx.

Leadership change. Changing the culture of a health care organization must start from the top. Every leader in the organization—executives, board members, senior management, and physician and nurse leaders—must share the same mission and goal for high reliability: eliminating harm completely. Leadership's commitment is the foundation upon which ultimate success rests.[6]

The leadership components in the framework are the following:

- ***Board:*** The board must play a prominent role in progressing toward zero patient harm by elevating quality and patient safety to the organization's highest strategic goal
- ***CEO/management:*** These leaders must move from an exclusive focus on regulatory compliance and toward the unified goal of zero patient harm.

- ***Physician involvement:*** Physicians must lead as well as participate in quality improvement throughout the organization.
- ***Quality strategy:*** Leaders must focus their organization's strategy to achieve high reliability, refining the organization's mission, values, and vision to focus on quality and safety and eliminate competing priorities.
- ***Quality measures:*** Quality must be measured and the resulting data must be widely available both with the hospital and to the public.
- ***Information technology (IT):*** Leaders must ensure that IT supporting quality improvement is coordinated and integrated into the organization's systems at a fundamental level.

The leadership stages of maturity related to these components are found in Figure 2-3 on the following page.

Call to Action

Leadership Change

Board members should commit to high reliability principles and follow through with actions that serve as an example to the entire staff, particularly when it comes to change and responding to it. Health care is a complex, constantly changing system. Resilient organizations are those that anticipate changes in risks and adapt accordingly. Governance and leadership must ensure that their organizations are engineered to be resilient to sustain quality efforts toward zero harm despite changing risks.[7]

Safety culture change. Since 2009, The Joint Commission has required leadership to create and maintain a culture of safety. This has been a challenge in many organizations. The Joint Commission also requires organizations to conduct staff surveys to assess the safety culture, but relatively few organizations utilize this data in productive ways.[6] Yet, high reliability rests squarely on the ability of an organization to inspire all staff members to make safety their top priority, and empower them to act when needed; therefore, safety culture is a critical, integral component.

FIGURE 2-3: Leadership and High Reliability: Stages of Organizational Maturity

LEADERSHIP	Beginning	Developing	Advancing	Approaching
Board	Board's quality focus is nearly exclusively on regulatory compliance.	Full board involvement in quality is limited to hearing reports from its quality committee.	Full board is engaged in development of quality goals and approval of a quality plan, and regularly reviews adverse events and progress on quality goals.	Board commits to the goal of high reliability (zero patient harm) for all clinical services.
CEO/ management	CEO/management's quality focus is nearly exclusively on regulatory compliance.	CEO acknowledges need for plan to improve quality and delegates the development and implementation of a plan to a subordinate.	CEO leads the development and implementation of a proactive quality agenda.	Management aims for zero patient harm for all vital clinical processes; some demonstrate zero or near-zero rates of harm.
Physician involvement	Physicians rarely lead quality improvement activities; overall participation by physicians in these activities is low.	Physicians champion some quality improvement activities; physicians participate in these activities in some areas, but not widely.	Physicians often lead quality improvement activities; physicians participate in these activities in most areas, but some important gaps remain.	Physicians routinely lead clinical quality improvement activities and accept the leadership of other appropriate clinicians; physicians' participation in these activities is uniform throughout the organization.
Quality strategy	Quality isn't identified as a central strategic imperative.	Quality is one of many competing strategic priorities.	Quality is one of the organization's top three or four strategic priorities.	Quality is the organization's highest-priority strategic goal.
Quality measures	Quality measures aren't prominently displayed nor reported internally or publicly; the only measures used are those required by outside entities and are not part of reward systems.	Few quality measures are reported internally; few or none are reported publicly and are not part of reward systems.	Routine internal reporting of quality measures begins, with the first measures reported publicly and the first quality metrics introduced into staff reward systems.	Key quality measures are routinely displayed internally and reported publicly; reward systems for staff prominently reflect the accomplishment of quality goals.
Information technology (IT)	IT provides little or no support for quality improvement.	IT supports some improvement activities, but principles of safe adoption are not often followed.	IT solutions support many quality initiatives; the organization commits to principles and the practice of safe adoption.	Safely adopted IT solutions are integral to sustaining improved quality.

Source: Chassin M, Loeb L. High-reliability health care: Getting there from here. *Milbank Q.* 2013 Sep;91(3):459–490. Accessed Aug 27, 2016. https://www.ncbi.nlm.nih.gov/pmc/articles/PMC3790522/pdf/milq0091-0459.pdf.

The safety culture components in the framework are the following:

- ***Trust:*** Organizations must establish trust, which grows when intimidating behavior is eliminated, reported problems are addressed quickly, and improvements are communicated to those who reported the problem.
- ***Accountability:*** Organizations must foster trust by holding all employees and medical staff accountable for prioritizing safety, and by applying a clear and fair system for separating blameless errors from those caused by reckless actions—with blameless errors treated as learning opportunities, while consistent disciplinary actions address cases of recklessness.
- ***Identifying unsafe conditions:*** Organizations must be proactive (rather than reactive when harm has already occurred) by identifying and addressing problems—including close calls and unsafe conditions—before they cause harm.
- ***Strengthening systems:*** Organizations must analyze data for many events to identify common systems that are causing problems (for example, infection control) instead of basing improvements on individual events.
- ***Assessment:*** Organizations must ensure that progress toward a safety culture is measured, analyzed, and improved just like any other PI project.

The safety culture stages of maturity related to these components are found in Figure 2-4 on the next page.

Robust Process Improvement. Process improvement is a series of actions to identify, analyze, and improve processes within an organization to meet new goals and objectives. Process improvement is achieved only with the right tools. The Center promotes use of a blended tool set—Lean Thinking, Six Sigma, and formal change management—as the most effective way to dramatically increase an organization's ability to approach zero patient harm. This initiative is known as Robust Process Improvement (RPI).

Briefly, the three tool sets used in RPI are as follows[6,8]:

- ***Lean Thinking:*** Focuses on customer satisfaction by way of increasing value and reducing wasted time, resources, and money
- ***Six Sigma:*** Measures a process for potential defects and helps organizations to eliminate variation by means of a statistical model
- ***Change management:*** Uses principles designed to increase the success and accelerate the implementation of organizational change efforts through ensuring accountability and acceptance

FIGURE 2-4: Safety Culture and High Reliability: Stages of Organizational Maturity

SAFETY CULTURE	Beginning	Developing	Advancing	Approaching
Trust	Trust or intimidating behavior is not assessed.	First codes of behavior are adopted in some clinical departments.	CEO and clinical leaders establish a trusting environment for all staff by modeling appropriate behaviors and championing efforts to eradicate intimidating behaviors.	High levels of (measured) trust exist in all clinical areas; self-policing of codes of behavior is in place.
Accountability	Emphasis is on blame; discipline is not applied equitably or with transparent standards; no process exists for distinguishing "blameless" from "blameworthy" acts.	The importance of equitable disciplinary procedures is recognized, and some clinical departments adopt these procedures.	Managers at all levels accord high priority to establishing all elements of safety culture; adoption of uniform equitable and transparent disciplinary procedures begins across the organization.	All staff recognize and act on their personal accountability for maintaining a culture of safety; equitable and transparent disciplinary procedures are fully adopted across the organization.
Identifying unsafe conditions	Root cause analysis is limited to adverse events; close calls ("early warnings") are not recognized or evaluated.	Pilot "close call" reporting programs begin in a few areas; some examples of early intervention to prevent harm can be found.	Staff in many areas begin to recognize and report unsafe conditions and practices before they harm patients.	"Close calls" and unsafe conditions are routinely reported, leading to early problem resolution before patients are harmed; results are routinely communicated.
Strengthening systems	Limited or no efforts exist to assess system defenses against quality failures and to remedy weaknesses.	Root cause analyses begin to identify the same weaknesses in system defenses in many clinical areas, but systematic efforts to strengthen them are lacking.	System weaknesses are cataloged and prioritized for improvement.	System defenses are proactively assessed, and weaknesses are proactively repaired.
Assessment	No measures of safety culture exist.	Some measures of safety culture are undertaken but are not widespread; little if any attempt is made to strengthen safety culture.	Measures of safety culture are adopted and deployed across the organization; efforts to improve safety culture are beginning.	Safety culture measures are part of the strategic metrics reported to the board; systematic improvement initiatives are under way to achieve a fully functioning safety culture.

Source: Chassin M, Loeb L. High-reliability health care: Getting there from here. *Milbank Q.* 2013 Sep;91(3):459–490. Accessed Aug 27, 2016. https://www.ncbi.nlm.nih.gov/pmc/articles/PMC3790522/pdf/milq0091-0459.pdf.

The three identified components of RPI are the following[6]:

- ***Methods:*** Organizations must utilize the full suite of tools offered by RPI as the formal approach to quality improvement
- ***Training:*** Organizations must aim to train every staff member and practitioner on RPI methods, as appropriate to their jobs.
- ***Spread:*** Organizations must use RPI tools across the organization for all improvement work and engage patients in redesigning care processes.

The RPI stages of maturity related to these components are found in Figure 2-5 on the next page.

High Reliability: Looking Forward

These changes in leadership, safety culture, and process improvement cannot happen overnight. Organizations should begin by assessing their current state of maturity for each component using the Oro 2.0 tool mentioned above. The Joint Commission is currently working on resources and tools to help leaders perform this assessment. As organizations begin to progress toward high reliability, their experiences will inform future efforts, guide development of resources, and become the basis for evaluating the framework's effectiveness.

The Next Step

As explained in this chapter, The Joint Commission is a valuable ally for organizations and their boards. Its methods, resources, and initiatives all support ever-higher levels of quality care. Chapter 3 offers practical suggestions and case study examples boards can use to serve their organizations and become effective leaders in the pursuit of quality and safety.

FIGURE 2-5: RPI and High Reliability: Stages of Organizational Maturity

ROBUST PROCESS IMPROVEMENT	Beginning	Developing	Advancing	Approaching
Methods	Organization has not adopted a formal approach to quality management.	Exploration of modern process improvement tools begins.	Organization commits to adopt the full suite of Robust Process Improvement (RPI) tools.	Adoption of RPI tools is accepted fully throughout the organization.
Training	Training is limited to compliance personnel or to the quality department.	Training in RPI tools outside the quality department is recognized as critical to success.	Training of selected staff in RPI is under way, and a plan is in place to broaden training.	Training in RPI is mandatory for all staff, as appropriate to their jobs.
Spread	No commitment to widespread adoption of improvement methods exists.	Pilot projects using some new tools are conducted in a few areas.	RPI is used in many areas to improve business processes as well as clinical quality and safety; a positive return on investment is achieved.	RPI tools are used throughout the organization for all improvement work; patients are engaged in redesigning care processes, and RPI proficiency is required for career advancement.

Source: Chassin M, Loeb L. High-reliability health care: Getting there from here. *Milbank Q.* 2013 Sep;91(3):459–490. Accessed Aug 27, 2016. https://www.ncbi.nlm.nih.gov/pmc/articles/PMC3790522/pdf/milq0091-0459.pdf.

REFERENCES

1. The Joint Commission. About The Joint Commission. Accessed Aug 27, 2016. http://www.jointcommission.org/about_us/about_the_joint_commission_main.aspx.
2. The Lewin Group. The value of Joint Commission accreditation for hospitals (unpublished consultation results). Jun 2012.
3. Wagner LM, McDonald SM, Castle NG. Relationship between nursing home safety culture and Joint Commission accreditation. *Jt Comm J Qual Patient Saf.* 2012 May;38(5):207–215.
4. Williams SC, et al. Comparing public quality ratings for accredited and nonaccredited nursing homes. *J Amer Med Dir Assoc.* 2016 Sep; 0(0). Accessed Sep 7, 2016. http://www.jamda.com/article/S1525-8610(16)30303-6/fulltext.
5. Pardini-Kiely K, et al. Improving and sustaining core measure performance through effective accountability of clinical microsystems in an academic medical center. *Jt Comm J Qual Patient Saf.* 2010 Sep;36(9):387–398.
6. Megan McHugh, PhD, et al. An early look at performance on the emergency care measures included in Medicare's hospital inpatient value-based purchasing program. *Ann Emerg Med.* 2013 Mar; (61)(6). 616–623.
7. Chassin MR, Loeb JM. High-reliability health care: Getting there from here. *Milbank Q.* 2013 Sep;91(3):459–490.
8. Blouin AS, McDonagh KJ. A framework for patient safety, part 2: Resilience, the next frontier. *J Nurs Adm.* 2011 Nov;41(11):450–452.

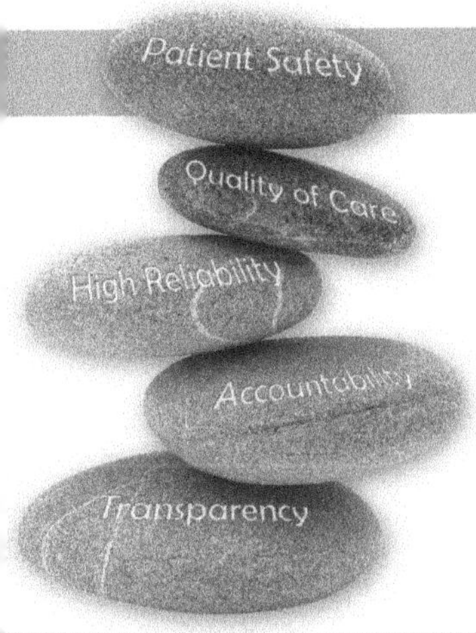

Chapter 3

The Board's Role in Improving Quality and Safety

In the ever-changing world of health care, the role of the board member may seem difficult to completely define. Many diverse issues need leadership attention: escalating costs, increased competition, changing regulatory requirements, increasing demand for better and safer care, and corporate pressure for better profitability. As discussed in Chapters 1 and 2, board members like yourself need to understand and take accountability for your medical, legal, and fiduciary responsibilities and determine how best to meet them. Fiduciary responsibility, remember, includes ultimate accountability not only for your organization's financial health but also for quality and safety performance; payment tied to quality and safety performance and customer satisfaction can have a major impact on financial health.

This chapter discusses ways that you and the rest of the board can make quality and safety a priority, including the following:

Board Engagement in Quality and Safety
- Putting Quality and Safety at the Top of the Board Agenda
- Creating a Board-Level Quality and Safety Committee
- Engaging the Board in Patient-Centered Activities

Board Accountability in Organizational Duties
- Encouraging Accountability via Transparency
- Promoting Leadership Accountability Through Evaluation
- Providing Incentives for Accountability
- Clarifying Leadership Accountability for Change
- Ensuring Collaboration for Accountability

Board Participation in PI
- Focusing on System Information for PI
- Determining PI Priorities and Allocating Resources
- Monitoring PI Results
- Using Dashboards to Oversee PI
- Submitting Written Reports on PI

Board Awareness of Regulations
- Joint Commission Requirements
- CMS Conditions
- Other Government Regulations

Development of a Multidisciplinary Board
- Seeking Physician Leadership and Insight
- Valuing Nurse Experience and Adaptability
- Recognizing Pharmacist Expertise and Management

Development of an Effective Board
- Governing vs. Managing
- Admitting Limitations
- Trusting and Communicating

Development of a Learning Board
- Bringing in a Quality and Safety Expert
- Listening to Frontline Staff
- Soliciting Patient Testimonials
- Finding Additional Learning Opportunities

Board Engagement in Quality and Safety

The impact boards have on quality and safety is not just a theory. A 2015 study has shown that hospitals with boards that pay greater attention to quality and safety have management that performs well in monitoring quality.[1] The importance of board leadership is a concept that most people know; however, that concept must be translated into practical actions to have a positive impact on quality and safety.[2] That concept and its practical application is addressed by Joint Commission and Centers for Medicare & Medicaid Services (CMS) requirements, which state that leadership—including boards—are ultimately responsible for the quality and safety provided at their organizations. This responsibility can be executed in many ways. Some common methods described below should be considered.

Putting Quality and Safety at the Top of the Board Agenda

Boards have a limited amount of time to spend on any one topic, so quality and safety must be scheduled high up on the agenda to ensure that these topics receive appropriate attention. Ideally, these discussions should go at the top of the agenda. Putting quality and safety at the top of the agenda can send a clear message to both management and administration that priorities have shifted, particularly if a board has traditionally given most of its time to fiscal matters. *See* Case Study: Restructuring the Board to Prioritize Safety (page 110) to learn how one hospital prioritized quality over finances and other issues.

Creating a Board-Level Quality and Safety Committee

Getting quality and safety on the board agenda can also be accomplished in other ways. An effective board utilizes a well-structured committee system to maximize its time and efficiency, and many boards establish a subcommittee or group dedicated to reviewing only quality and safety issues. The committee may include board members, senior organization leaders, department directors, and/or patient and family representatives.

Reports on quality and safety. Quality and safety should not just stay in a committee; the entire board needs to understand the organization's performance in these areas. But a board-level quality and safety committee can help address key challenges and sort through management reports for information that's relevant and necessary to pass along to the whole board. Written reports to, by, and between the board and its quality and safety committee are, in fact, the cornerstone of quality and safety oversight. These include recent patient safety events as well as information on the organization's performance compared to its own past performance, the performance of similar organizations in other parts of the country, and comparison to relevant standards and regulations, including those for Joint Commission accreditation. Understanding how the organization performs on accreditation and certification surveys is a key oversight function. And, of course, reporting must rest firmly upon a culture of safety, with transparency and respect of utmost importance.

Goals and action plans for quality and safety. The quality and safety committee not only focuses the organization's approach to quality and safety but

continued on page 113

• CASE STUDY •

Restructuring the Board to Prioritize Safety

WHO THEY ARE

Massachusetts General Hospital in Boston is the third oldest general hospital in the United States. Its 999-bed facility admits approximately 48,000 inpatients, handles nearly 1.5 million outpatient visits, and records more than 100,000 emergency room visits every year.

WHAT THEY DID

When the Institute of Medicine issued its report *Crossing the QualityChasm: A New Health System for the 21st Century in 2001* (*see* Chapter 1), Massachusetts General was inspired to undertake a major organizational shift. The hospital unified its diffuse quality and safety efforts into a single cultural focus, directed by the board.

Centralization. Under the prior system, the hospital's safety initiatives were undertaken by individual units or departments. While these did improve care, the lack of centralized coordination and inadequate communications resulted in inefficiencies. Many cases of redundant efforts occurred, such as collecting the same data several times for different purposes. Confusion about roles and responsibilities was also present, which negatively impacted accountability.

Centralizing quality and safety directed by the board meant that board members would have to devote more time to those issues than they'd previously done. To do so, the board members, who had strong business backgrounds, needed to be as fluent on quality and safety issues as they were on finance. Similarly, all levels of leadership throughout the hospital needed to be involved in this new focus on safety.

Education and incentives. To this end, the hospital organized a series of executive educational retreats. Special effort was given to engaging middle management, as these individuals hadn't previously been a part of safety and quality efforts. To build accountability, the incentive system at Massachusetts General was adjusted to include rewards for quality achievements. The quality incentives became equivalent to financial incentives, which both encouraged improvement and also demonstrated just how seriously the hospital was taking quality and safety.

THEIR RESULTS

Shifting its board structure to a quality and safety focus has had several effects. The board now spends more time talking about safety and quality issues than financial ones. All meetings lead off with a quality and safety update presented by the hospital's CEO. This practice demonstrates to the board that the CEO is invested in these issues, knows what's happening inside the organization concerning quality and safety challenges, and is dedicated to improvement.

Successes as well as failures. Also, the board's safety and quality discussions have begun to incorporate instances of both failure and success. It's important to know where the organization has fallen short, but it recognizes that it's equally important to know what it did that was right.

Patient stories. Achieving and maintaining the board's enthusiasm for safety is due in part to the increasing use of patient stories and personal anecdotes in board discussions. The primary benefit of anecdotes, the organization discovered, is making the issues real to the board members. For example, in the course of discussing hand hygiene rates, it was mentioned that better hand hygiene was linked to decreased rates of methicillin-resistant staphylococcus aureus (MRSA) and vancomycin-resistant enterococci (VRE) infections. One board member spoke up and shared that a family member developed a MRSA infection elsewhere, and described what it was like for the patient and the family.

Patient stories related from the patients themselves are also an important resource. Massachusetts General has invited several patients to speak about their experiences at board meetings, and plans to do so more frequently in the future.

Hard questions. Gauging the level of board investment in safety issues can be tricky. Leaders observe that the board is "on board" when they ask hard questions. Challenging questions from board members are an indication that they care enough about the issues to have high expectations. The leaders also want the board to hold staff and providers accountable, determining that those individuals will be inspired to do a better job if they know the board members will be examining the reports closely and asking questions. The organization noted that when the safety questions are as hard as the financial ones, you know you're there.

SIDEBAR 3-1

Creating an Effective Quality and Safety Committee

Many organizations have a board-level quality and safety committee, but without proper oversight, the committee might not be successful. Effective committees of this type typically do the following:

Look beyond the minimum: The quality and safety committee should strive to go beyond the basic requirements or industry averages. It should prioritize improvements based on opportunities for performance excellence, setting goals based on the most critical issues and challenges that will provide the highest return on investment of time and resources, which usually means focusing on high-risk areas.

Utilize diverse perspectives: A multidisciplinary group is best. The quality and safety committee should be composed of experts in clinical improvement, safety, process improvement tools, and patient experience. These individuals may be from within the organization or from external organizations.

Educate themselves: Keeping up to date on trends, performance standards, and improvement approaches is critical. A quality and safety committee that's continually seeking to improve its knowledge base is one that can keep its board and organization ahead of the change curve.

Prioritize improvements and allocate resources accordingly: As organizations improve, patient populations shift, and regulations change; thus the needs of the organization also change. Quality and safety committees should regularly review the organization's performance, identify opportunities for improvement, and make sure that those projects get the staff and financial support they need to succeed.

Hold themselves and others accountable: The quality and safety committee can take on the task of assessing the performance of itself, the board, and organization leadership in achieving improvement goals. One method is to ask clinical and administrative leaders to update the committee several times a year. This is a way to motivate leaders to improve and provide guidance or assistance in cases where improvement is lacking.

Source: Byrnes J. Using the board quality committee to drive the value proposition. *Healthc Financ Manage.* 2014 Aug;68(8):92–93.

also champions the integration of this approach throughout the organization and oversees the performance improvement (PI) process. This means developing action plans that engage the individuals and departments responsible for PI activities. For example, the quality and safety committee may direct the organization's infection control committee to investigate why there's been a rise in health care–associated infections (HAIs). The board committee should then receive ongoing updates on the progress of action plans addressing such quality and safety challenges. (Board involvement in performance measurement and improvement will be discussed in greater detail later in this chapter.) Sidebar 3-1 on page 112 provides some guidance on this type of committee.

Engaging the Board in Patient-Centered Activities

Perhaps one of the most important ways board members can make time for quality and safety is to "leave the board room." In other words, you and the rest of the board should take part in activities that bring you into contact with patients and staff.

Participation in patient-centered activities has several benefits. First, it helps break down the invisible barriers between leaders and frontline staff, which in turn encourages communication and supports the culture of safety (as described in Chapters 1 and 2). These activities also provide board members with valuable insights and perspectives they can't get from a report or spreadsheet. Seeing the everyday challenges to safety that confront patients and staff makes those challenges real for board members, who may not have a clinical background or understand how policy translates into practice.

WalkRounds™ and shadowing. A WalkRound is exactly what it sounds like: a walk around the organization, visiting various areas and talking to staff members about quality and safety issues. Developed by the Institute for Healthcare Improvement (IHI) and Allan Frankel, MD, it involves senior leaders touring a unit or department at least weekly to (1) demonstrate quality and safety as a high organizational priority and (2) engage in informal discussions with direct care staff about patient safety issues. It's a commonly used tool for identifying improvement opportunities as well. The flowchart in Figure 3-1 on page 114 shows how it works for unit-based rounds. Board members may want to join these WalkRounds. Any discussions should begin by stressing that there will be no reprisals or blame directed at those who report patient safety events and that safety is everyone's responsibility and highest priority. Asking open-ended questions lets the staff know that leadership takes safety issues seriously and is willing to listen to their concerns.

FIGURE 3-1: WalkRounds™

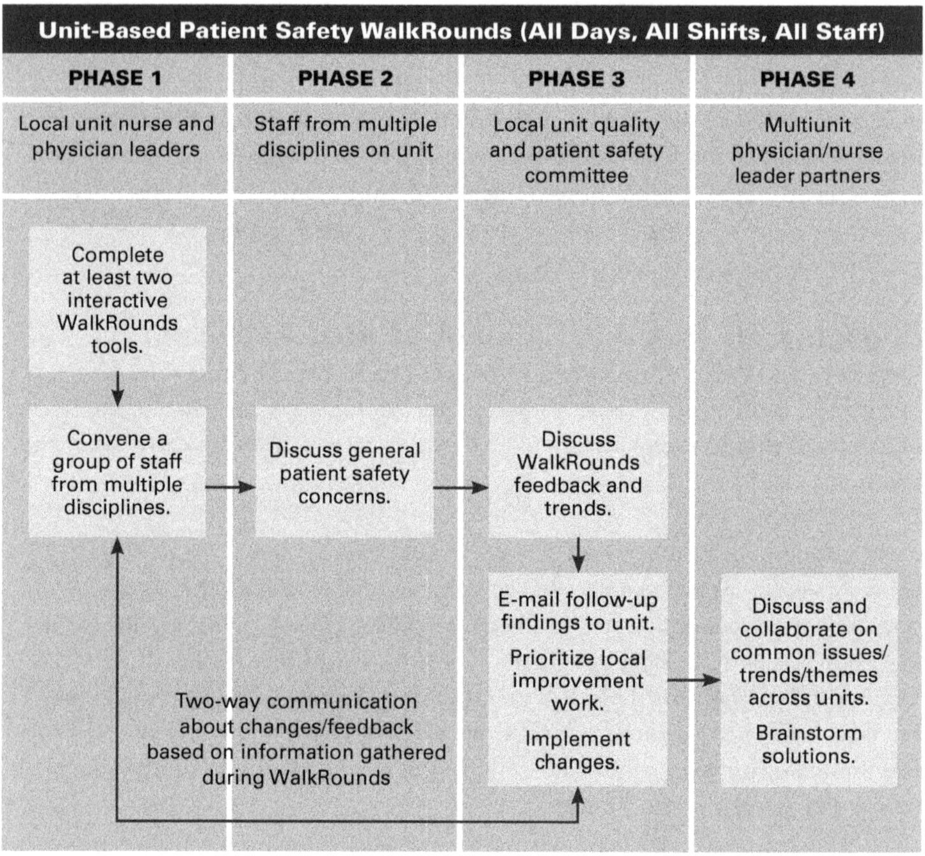

The phases are as follows: **Phase 1:** Local nurse and physician leaders convene a group of frontline staff and complete a short safety assessment for the unit. **Phase 2:** Leaders engage the group in a general discussion of patient safety concerns. **Phase 3:** Leaders discuss findings with the local unit quality and safety committee. **Phase 4:** Leaders discuss findings with unit leaders across units to identify macro-level safety issues.

The WalkRounds tool is available from the Institute for Healthcare Improvement on its website: www.ihi.org/resources/pages/tools/patientsafetyleadershipwalkrounds.aspx.

Similarly, boards may want to establish a shadowing program. Following a physician or other clinician through his or her daily routine provides board members with yet another valuable perspective.

WalkRounds and shadowing activities should be documented, including topics discussed, contributing factors for each issue, and possible follow-up actions. Documentation provides a record of the experience that supports accountability and continued monitoring of challenges facing the organization.

Quality and safety initiatives. Board members may want to sponsor or otherwise become involved in a particular quality and safety initiative. Sometimes, these arise from a WalkRound or shadowing experience. Or, it may be that a board member relates to an issue in a personal way or has background in a subject. For example, you may be particularly interested in improving medication safety, preventing HAIs in the intensive care unit, or meeting federal requirements for Medicare reimbursement.

Other ways to get involved in patient-centered care. As long as there are no conflicts of interest, these situations can be great learning experiences for board members and present opportunities to share knowledge and experience. A leader's passion or interest in a topic is contagious. It can inspire others to become similarly dedicated to the initiative or project.

Other ways you and other board members can get involved with patient-centered care include the following:

- ***Invite staff to speak at a board meeting:*** Ask staff members working in an area that needs improvement to speak at a quality and safety committee or board meeting. Their passion and insights are valuable and important for the board to witness.
- ***Invite patients to speak at a board meeting:*** Ask former patients to share their care experiences with the board, either in person or through a video or written narrative. This kind of feedback is extremely valuable.
- ***Give kudos to those who earn it:*** Visit an area of the organization that has made great strides in quality or safety to congratulate staff members on their achievements and encourage progress elsewhere.

Call to Action
Making Board Time for Quality and Safety

Understanding the critical role board members can play in quality and safety improvement is an essential component of board education. Orientation early and often to emerging quality and safety challenges makes a board more knowledgeable and helps the board really govern. And engaging in quality and safety activities can support informed decision making, a strong culture of safety, and ultimately improve patient safety and quality of care. As a start, read your organization's policies, maybe one per month: Does each one clearly state goals related to quality and safety? Does the documentation required support risk assessment and performance measurement? If not, take time to improve these policies with the help of the rest of the organization leaders and staff.

Board Accountability in Organizational Duties

As you learned in Chapter 1, boards are increasingly accountable to many different groups: accrediting organizations, regulatory authorities, government agencies, the public, and so on. Board members must understand, demonstrate, and monitor how well they are fulfilling their duties to these various groups and providing what's promised.

Encouraging Organizational Accountability via Transparency

The importance of transparency and honest communication has been stressed throughout this book, and with good reason. Transparency to the public of your organization's quality and safety performance data is expected in today's market. Transparency is also the key to developing a proactive safety culture and is an underlying component of high reliability organizations, as noted in Chapter 2. Boards need to recognize that an effective safety culture will expose process defects, and those defects are opportunities for learning and improvement. Organizations should seek out these process failures rather than avoid them. All staff members should feel responsible for, and be encouraged to participate in, maintaining high-quality, safe care. They should know they're expected to identify and address problems without worrying about "how things look."

The National Patient Safety Foundation's (NPSF) Lucian Leape Institute offers discussion on the importance of health care transparency, and guidance on how to achieve it.[3] Its 2015 report, *Shining a Light: Safer Health Care Through Transparency*, can be downloaded on the NPSF website: www.npsf.org/?shiningalight.

Promoting Leadership Accountability Through Evaluation

One way to promote leadership accountability is to incorporate quality and safety goals into senior leaders' and midlevel managers' annual performance evaluations. These goals will differ from one organization to another, but they should align with the overall strategic goals the board has approved. For example, goals may address clinical indicators such as ORYX® core measures (*see* Chapter 2), patient satisfaction, compliance with National Patient Safety Goals (NPSGs) (*see* Chapter 2), or provision of necessary staffing (*see* Chapter 1).

Board evaluations. Boards themselves need evaluation too. Self-assessment can identify leadership gaps that can be addressed with board succession planning. Boards that evaluate their own performance in a thorough, honest fashion may do the following[4]:

- Discover growth opportunities for existing board members.
- Recruit new trustees who fill gaps.
- Customize board education and training to meet the board's and the organization's unique needs.

To be effective, the board evaluation process should be clearly defined in writing, ideally in a policy operating procedure and/or bylaws. Important components include the following[5]:

- To whom the board is accountable, such as financial stakeholders, regulatory authorities, accrediting organizations such as The Joint Commission, and community groups
- Specific responsibilities of the board, its committees, and its members
- Description of actions necessary to implement the policy

Boards may want to develop metrics to assess how well they meet their responsibilities to those organizations to which they're accountable. These can be assembled into a dashboard, just like any other compliance data, and used to monitor performance and identify areas for improvement. Dashboards and metrics are discussed later in this chapter.

Call to Action
Board Evaluations

The concept of what makes a good board member is changing. Today, the ideal board member must bring more to the boardroom than financial know-how. Many organizations now select and evaluate board members based on a set of competencies. These lists of skills can be used as tools for both recruitment of new members and evaluation of existing ones. The competencies should be reviewed periodically to ensure that they still reflect the organization's needs. They should also be revisited after a major organizational change, such as a merger or an acquisition, or an addition of new clinical services.

Providing Incentives for Accountability

Financial incentives are a common method of encouraging performance through competition. As organizations and their boards are increasingly accountable for safety and quality, so too must incentives reflect performance on safety and quality metrics.

Incentives for executive accountability. Despite the cultural shift toward quality in recent years, quality metrics are still not consistently used in determining financial incentives. This is changing, but slowly. Nonprofit organizations are increasingly using quality incentives in compensation for top executives. According to one survey, two thirds of nonprofit hospitals included quality metrics in executive incentives in 2013, up from 57% the previous year and 45% five years before that.[6] Though far from universal, linking executive incentives to quality metrics is trending upward. This is a direct reflection of the Affordable Care Act (ACA) value-based reimbursement system, which puts pressure on health care organizations to improve quality. In some cases, pay is being linked to population health as well (*see* Chapter 1).[7]

Boards of all organizations should find a balance between base salaries and incentives for executives. Quality-based incentives should, for example, be based on appropriate performance metrics that are aligned with the organization's goals and regulatory requirements.[7] If a health care organization has never before linked quality and safety to executive performance, the board may need to introduce changes to bonus payments by degrees. As the organizational culture becomes more focused on quality and safety, leaders will be more likely to agree with and even promote the move away from solely finance-based metrics.

Incentives for staff accountability. The need for organizationwide ownership of quality and safety has been emphasized throughout this book. If this is to be accomplished, quality and safety measures should be included in staff incentives as well as executive incentives. Boards can support this by tying all employees' performance to quality and safety improvement. An important step is assessing each employee's ability to meet quality and safety goals at annual performance reviews.

Physicians, like organizations, now have their Medicare reimbursements tied to the quality of care they provide. Under the ACA, physicians who don't report satisfactory performance data to CMS will have their Medicare payments reduced.[8] The goal is to make physicians responsible for improving their own performance. You and other board members should keep these changes in mind when assessing the compensation for the physicians who are employed by your organization. This is especially important due to the increasing number of physicians who have become hospital or medical group employees in recent years, from 38% in 2008 to 53% in 2014.[9]

Clarifying Leadership Accountability for Change

The governing body is responsible for the performance of an entire organization. Therefore, it makes sense that the CEO and other senior leaders should be held responsible for helping the organization meet its performance goals. Some executives may feel that such accountability is unfair, given that their ability to achieve positive results depends in part on how much support they receive from the board. If trustees set unrealistic goals or refuse to provide the resources necessary to achieve goals, there's little chance that the CEO can effect required changes. To resolve this tension, it may be helpful to clarify the roles of executives and the board. For example, the CEO and senior leaders are responsible for daily operations, while the board is responsible for overall strategy and governance. The emphasis of accountability should be to gain executive commitment to help the organization deliver the best health care possible.

Managing change. Change can be difficult, especially the kind of large-scale, fundamental change necessary to adapt to the new health care culture. Leadership can make it easier, and more sustainable, by effectively managing the changes needed. Managing change requires that everyone at the organization, from frontline staff to top executives, understands the following[10]:

- ***What the change is:*** Saying "we need to create a culture of safety" is not enough. Leaders must use vivid, concrete reasoning to make sure staff members visualize the new environment.
- ***Why the change is important:*** Knowing the reason behind a change is a big part of getting people to fully commit to it.
- ***The consequences of not changing:*** People need to understand the organizational and personal impact if they fail to pursue the change laid out by the board and leadership.
- ***How the change will happen:*** People should be informed of the steps that will be taken, the goals along the way, and the time line to achieve them.
- ***How the change affects them:*** People want to know what their roles will be during and after the change is implemented. Making the change personal is critical to making it sustainable in the long term.

A healthy culture of safety, grounded in open communication and transparency, supports this process of managing change. People cannot be afraid of asking questions, making mistakes, or admitting their weaknesses, particularly during a time of change.

Ensuring Collaboration for Accountability

Effective boards and effective management are closely related, and both positively affect quality. Studies show that high-quality hospitals (that is, those that have high performance on clinical quality metrics) have both strong boards and strong management.[1] In addition, evidence indicates that maintaining positive, effective working relationships among leadership groups has a positive impact on organizational performance.[11] This should be a strong incentive for organizations to purposefully foster collaboration between the board and management and be accountable for maintaining that collaboration.

Inevitable conflict. Achieving and maintaining effective collaboration, however, can be a challenge. Conflict is inevitable, and even when leadership groups are unified under a single goal, there can be disagreement over interpretation of data and which actions will best meet that goal. Conflict itself is not necessarily bad; it can indicate that participants are actively, thoughtfully engaged in issues. But conflicts that are managed poorly, or arise from a weak or nonexistent culture of safety, will result in strained or ineffective working relationships.[12]

Collaboration strategies. Strategies to consider when thinking about improving board-management collaboration include the following:

- ***Clearly define roles, responsibilities, expectations, and boundaries:*** Boards are expected to be active participants in safety and quality, yet this can be, or be perceived to be, authoritarian or overly restrictive.[11] Boards and management alike must know what each group is responsible for, and equally important, what they are not. In general terms, management designs and implements processes, and the board encourages and motivates management to do so.[13] When one group fails to meet its responsibility, or attempts to do the other's job, the result is resentment and eroded trust. Managers should follow the board's guidance, but the board must not let their actions interfere too much with managers' autonomy or overstep directly into clinical matters.[11,13]
- ***Manage conflicts:*** Conflict management should begin before a conflict arises. The Joint Commission Leadership (LD) standards require leadership groups to work together to establish a clear process for handling conflicts quickly and in ways that don't compromise quality and safety. Individuals with conflict management skills will be very helpful in establishing and carrying out this process as well as helping you to avoid conflicts before they happen.[13]
- ***Establish appropriate flow of information:*** Working together requires communication. Information on quality and safety metrics, PI efforts, and changes to policy and procedure must flow freely among boards and management. Expectations and accountability related to reporting should be clearly set.[14]
- ***Reinforce safety culture:*** Board-management collaboration is yet another area supported by a strong safety culture. The tenets of transparency, trust, and open communication that create a culture of safety also underlie conflict management, information flow, and other aspects of working relationships. Boards and management must have trust and respect in order for any other collaboration strategy to be effective.

Board Participation in PI

Board members are ultimately accountable for the results of PI efforts even though they don't participate in day-to-day PI activities. And, as noted at the beginning of Chapter 1, as reimbursement rules shift to a pay-for-quality standard under the ACA, boards must make PI on quality and safety metrics their top priority. So, what exactly should the board do in regard to PI?

Focusing on System Information for PI

The board's role should focus on high-level, whole-system trends and related improvements. The tendency for management to provide so much information that boards get bogged down in details isn't helpful. If boards are presented with too much, or too complex, information, the "big picture" items and trends they need to know can be hard to pick out.[15]

This doesn't mean that review of individual measure data should be abandoned altogether. Those data just need to be selected carefully, with one metric (such as an organization's overall infection rate), to represent many contributing patient safety factors. A change in the large-scale number can indicate the need for a closer look.[16]

Determining PI Priorities and Allocating Resources

After reviewing data, the board must make decisions regarding priorities for PI and allocation of resources to support improvement efforts. To do this, it needs information that's accurate and relevant. Boards and management should feel comfortable asking questions of each other when there's confusion over a metric, or when more information is needed. Open communication, based on trust and fostered in a culture of safety, makes this possible.

Factors and questions. Factors helpful in making decisions about PI projects—and questions to ask about them—include the following:

- ***Experts:*** What are the suggestions from people who deal with performance gaps (quality and patient safety leaders, patient safety officers, medical directors, nurse leaders, other clinical leaders)?
- ***Themes:*** Do any systemic themes pop up in the data (communication, equipment and supplies, adverse events)?
- ***Reporting requirements:*** Are the reporting requirements for performance data on a project mandatory or elective, and what's involved?
- ***Performance gap history:*** Are previous or ongoing improvement efforts achieving their goals?

Monitoring PI Results

One of the most important aspects of any PI effort is monitoring the results of that effort. Has safety improved? Have goals been met? If not, what's going wrong, and what else could be done? Perhaps work stalled because more staff time was needed than originally projected. Or, perhaps the changes required a bigger cultural change than anticipated, meaning the goal will take longer to reach. In any case, the board needs to know what's happening with the organization's key initiatives.

Boards should ensure that they're armed with the latest information and can apply current approaches and concepts. This may mean keeping up to date on developments from The Joint Commission (such as revisions to the NPSGs or changes in ORYX performance measure requirements), CMS, the National Quality Forum, or the Agency for Healthcare Research and Quality. Boards may also want to monitor nationwide trends on issues that their organizations are currently targeting for improvement.

Conversation Starters
Board Participation in PI

- *What system-related improvement efforts are we engaged in presently?*
- *Are there sufficient resources for those efforts?*
- *How are we monitoring the results of those efforts?*
- *What are the results so far?*
- *Are we using the most current evidence-based approaches?*
- *What is the control plan for sustaining those improvements?*
- *What if the improvements are not sustained?*

As board members, you should also understand what kinds of information you're looking at as you monitor performance, and what that information means. Several different kinds of data are commonly used to measure performance.

Quantitative and qualitative data. First, as you probably know, there are two kinds of data: *Quantitative data* describe anything that can be counted and written down in numbers. One example is the number of discharged patients screened for and provided with the influenza vaccine if indicated. *Qualitative data* are often less concrete because they're based on perception and opinion. For example, patient satisfaction is a subjective concept, even if it is expressed with numerical value (for example, on a scale of 1 to 10).

Both quantitative and qualitative data have value to an organization. However, qualitative data should not be the sole basis for determining quality of care or PI. Rather, qualitative data can help interpret the "hard" numbers that indicate a weakness.[16] For example, an organization makes changes to its admissions process in an effort to improve patient flow and collect better patient history information. If patient surveys show dissatisfaction with the new process, the organization may want to look at it again to see what might be causing that perception. Perhaps a particular form is confusing to fill out, or the patients are unsure what health information they need to provide, or the new process takes longer and increases wait times.

Outcome measures and process measures. Organizations use two kinds of quantitative data measurements: outcome measures and process measures:

- ***Outcome measures:*** These assess the result of performance (or nonperformance) of a function or process and quantify the end results of health care. These end points include mortality, readmission rates, and health care–associated surgical site infection rates.
- ***Process measures:*** These assess the proportion of times that an indicated health care service was provided to patients. The performance rate on a process measure indicates how many times the organization was presented with the situation, and how often the indicated health care treatment or intervention was provided: for example, the percentage of patients aged 6 months and older seen for a visit between October 1, and March 31, who were screened for and received an influenza immunization if indicated.

Outcome measures can be useful to boards, as they provide the end results of care. But they don't give any information on *why* the rate is what it is—that's where process measures come in. How well an organization performs on process measures affects the outcome measures. Process measures must be granular to be useful to boards, unless they're presented as a potential target for improvement, or unless affected by an internal or external change, such as a new service being offered or a new regulation going into effect.

Using Dashboards to Oversee PI

To perform their duties regarding performance, whether setting priorities or monitoring progress, boards need accurate information presented in a way that's easy to understand. The most commonly used format is the dashboard.

Dashboards (sometimes called scorecards) can take many forms, but ultimately they're designed to display data in a visual way that's quickly and easily understandable. There's no right or wrong way to do this, and every organization's dashboard(s) will be different. This is both good and bad. It's good, because it means the dashboard format is flexible enough to adapt to most situations. The drawback is that no standards exist to ensure that the information on a particular dashboard is presented accurately and interpreted properly.

Standards for dashboard metrics. A study of safety and quality dashboards[17] found that the metrics included varied greatly and often provided an inaccurate view of the organization's performance. The study indicated that the large number of quality and safety measures included on dashboards suggests that boards are genuinely interested in these issues. However, the specific measures being represented frequently reflected efficiency, patient satisfaction, and productivity rather than quality and safety.[17] Further, outcome measures (which are often used on dashboards) don't have standardized thresholds and were in fact more useful at identifying hazards than measuring quality and safety.[17]

The study further suggests that boards should hold quality and safety reports to the same standard as financial reports. In other words, boards should insist that quality and safety reports be clear, focused, prioritized, based on defined measures, and compare previous internal and external reports and benchmarks.[17]

Strategies for creating dashboards. The following are some issues to keep in mind when designing effective, reliable dashboards—any of which can be suggested to those who develop dashboards to board members:

Put quality and safety first: An organization that puts quality and safety first should have a board that does the same. Every dashboard used by an organization should bring those issues to the front. Also, quality and safety should be incorporated into every dashboard, instead of being just one among many.[15]

Customize for various purposes: Different audiences have different needs. The board's quality and safety committee, for example, will need a greater level of detail than the whole board. Similarly, management may create a dashboard focused solely on current improvement projects, to update the board on progress.[15]

Select relevant, useful information: Strike a balance between high-level concepts and specific measures that are critical components of these concepts. For example, if the surgical site infection rate is trending downward, the dashboard might include performance data on related processes that are also trending downward. Any useful dashboard should include key performance indicators (KPIs).

Use visual cues carefully: Color-coding, stars, graphs, and other visual elements can make the dashboard easy to read. These must be used cautiously, though. Simplified grading systems like color coding can imply a false sense of quality. For example, many dashboards use green to indicate performance that meets standards. But what standards are they? Setting low goals may result in a uniformly green dashboard, but that does not mean the organization is performing well. To avoid this, organizations should be sure their performance indicators reflect appropriate goals.[15]

Build in adaptability: Dashboards should be frequently evaluated to determine whether they're still relevant and effective. As new areas of concern emerge, relevant metrics should be added to the dashboard. The dashboard should also be responsive to the changing needs of the board, as requested and appropriate.

The sample dashboard in Figure 3-2 on page 127 shows KPIs for select Joint Commission Environment of Care (EC) and Life Safety (LS) standards.

Conversation Starters
Using Dashboards to Oversee PI

- *Does our organization use dashboards to monitor PI?*
- *If so, do the measures reflect quality and safety?*
- *How often are they evaluated and adapted for new metrics and new needs?*

Submitting Written Reports on PI

Summary dashboards can be a convenient and efficient way of conveying information quickly. But sometimes an issue is complex and cannot be adequately expressed in a simplified format. Written reports may be a better way to build a case for a project's prioritization or budget review, for example. Narrative can provide guidance on interpretation of measures or give background information that provides context. Organizations might encourage their management teams to provide written reports that supplement their dashboards, where needed.

FIGURE 3-2: KPI Summary Dashboard

Environment of Care & Life Safety Key Performance Indicators

Standard	Description	1st Quarter Compliant	1st Quarter Non-compliant	2nd Quarter Compliant	2nd Quarter Non-compliant	3rd Quarter Compliant	3rd Quarter Non-compliant	4th Quarter Compliant	4th Quarter Non-compliant	Overall Compliance
EC.02.05.01	**The hospital manages risk associated with its utility systems.**	**76.54%**	**23.46%**	**74.56%**	**25.44%**	**64.26%**	**35.74%**	**77.20%**	**22.80%**	**73.14%**
LS.02.01.20	The hospital maintains the integrity of the means of egress.	98.70%	1.30%	96.23%	3.77%	95.36%	4.64%	99.48%	0.52%	97.44%
EC.02.06.01	**The hospital establishes and maintains a safe, functional environment.**	**93.68%**	**6.32%**	**96.61%**	**3.39%**	**91.50%**	**8.50%**	**94.39%**	**5.61%**	**94.05%**
EC.02.03.05	The hospital maintains fire safety equipment and fire safety building features.	100.00%	0.00%	98.75%	1.25%	97.59%	2.41%	99.32%	0.68%	98.92%
LS.02.01.10	Building and fire protection features are designed and maintained to minimize the effects of fire, smoke, and heat.	96.40%	3.60%	98.72%	1.28%	95.33%	4.67%	98.72%	1.28%	97.29%
LS.02.01.30	**The hospital provides and maintains building features to protect individuals from the hazards of fire and smoke.**	**96.19%**	**3.81%**	**93.65%**	**6.35%**	**89.05%**	**10.95%**	**95.99%**	**4.01%**	**93.72%**
LS.02.01.35	**The hospital provides and maintains systems for extinguishing fires.**	**93.68%**	**6.32%**	**96.61%**	**3.39%**	**91.50%**	**8.50%**	**94.39%**	**5.61%**	**94.05%**
EC.02.02.01	The hospital manages risks related to hazardous materials and waste.	98.77%	1.23%	98.77%	1.23%	96.53%	3.47%	95.04%	4.96%	97.28%
EC.02.05.09	The hospital inspects, tests, and maintains medical gas and vacuum systems.	100.00%	0.00%	99.35%	0.65%	100.00%	0.00%	98.93%	1.07%	99.57%
EC.02.05.07	The hospital inspects, tests, and maintains emergency power systems.	99.53%	0.47%	98.12%	1.88%	100.00%	0.00%	98.12%	1.88%	98.94%

***Bolded standards are examples of non-compliance for an organization with a goal of 95% or greater.**

Standard	Compliance Percentage	Non-Compliance Percentage
EC.02.05.01 Utility Mgmt	76.54%	23.46%
LS.02.01.20 Egress	97.44%	2.56%
EC.02.06.01 Safe & Functional Environment	94.05%	5.96%
EC.02.03.05 Fire Safety Equipment	98.92%	1.09%
LS.02.01.10 Fire Safety Design	97.29%	2.71%
LS.02.01.30 Fire Safety Maintenance	93.72%	6.28%
LS.02.01.35 Extinguishment	94.05%	5.96%
EC.02.02.01 Hazmat	97.28%	2.72%
EC.02.05.09 Medical Gas & Vacuum	99.57%	0.43%
EC.02.05.07 Emergency Power	98.94%	1.06%
Environment of Care	94.21%	5.79%
Life Safety	95.63%	4.38%

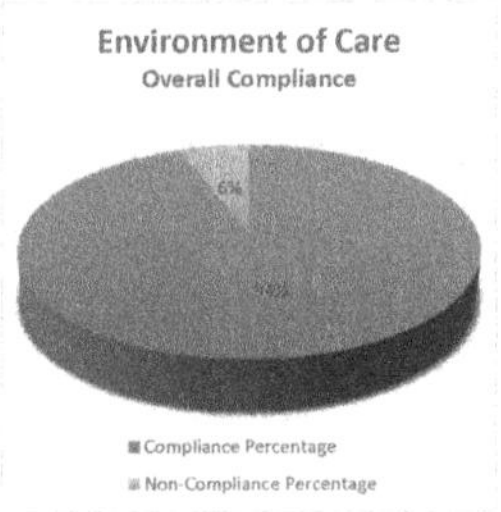

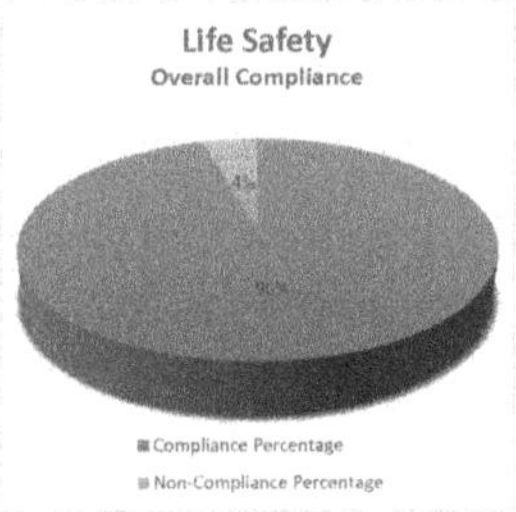

This dashboard provides an overview of the key performance indicators (KPIs) in a hospital's physical environment. The KPIs are Environment of Care (EC) and Life Safety (LS) standards that the organization has chosen to include in their compliance analysis.

Joint Commission written report requirements. The Joint Commission, realizing the value of written reports, requires a number of such reports be submitted to leadership on a regular basis. This includes, for hospitals and critical access hospitals, a written report of data analysis results on issues related to adequacy of staffing for annual review by leaders responsible for your patient safety program. Written reports for board review and approval, which include those for PI, are listed in the checklist in Figure 3-3 on page 129.

These reports are often the basis for discussion among leadership on issues that affect the organization and the population(s) it serves, including the following:

- Performance improvement activities
- Reported safety and quality issues
- Proposed solutions and their impact on the organization's resources
- Reports on key quality measures and safety indicators
- Safety and quality issues specific to the population(s) served
- Input from the population(s) served

Leaders act on or comply with these internal reports as well as reports and recommendations from external agencies, such as accreditation, certification, or regulatory bodies, which is briefly addressed in the next section.

Board Awareness of Regulations

Requirements for written reports to leadership are just one type of requirement among many related to quality and safety. It's impossible to know every one of them, but it's important to grasp the range of requirements and regulations in this area that are issued from various sources, including The Joint Commission, CMS, and other authorities.

Joint Commission Requirements

As discussed in Chapter 2, Joint Commission accreditation is determined by an organization's compliance with Joint Commission standards and other requirements, including performance measure submission and National Patient Safety Goals. All accredited and certified organizations have complimentary access to E-dition®, the electronic repository for the applicable Joint Commission requirements for their particular organization. The same requirements can be accessed in a hard-copy comprehensive accreditation manual, which can be purchased.

FIGURE 3-3: Required Board Review and Approval Checklist

Required Board Review and Approval Checklist
Accreditation Programs/Settings: AHC, BHC, CAH, HAP, LAB, NCC, OBS, OME

Required Board Review and Approval Checklist

This checklist includes documents that need to be submitted to your board (or other governing body) for review or approval, per Joint Commission standards. Most are documents that require board approval when initiated or modified. You can use it to make sure that you have the governance involvement as required.

Organization: ______________________________

Date of Review: ____________ Reviewer: ______________________________

Annual Written Reports from Leadership *(board review)* [AHC, BHC, CAH, HAP, NCC, OME]

✔ N/A
- ☐ ☐ System or process failures
- ☐ ☐ Number and type of sentinel events
- ☐ ☐ Whether patients and families were informed of the event
- ☐ ☐ All actions taken to improve safety, both proactively and in response to events
- ☐ ☐ Determined number of distinct improvement projects to be conducted annually [HAP for deemed status only]
- ☐ ☐ Results of analyses related to adequacy of staff

Human Resources *(board approval)* [CAH, HAP]

✔ N/A
- ☐ ☐ Equivalent process for credentialing and privileging physician assistants and advanced practice registered nurses

Medical Staff *(board approval)* [CAH, HAP]

✔ N/A
- ☐ ☐ Structure of the organized medical staff (if applicable) [CAH only to rehabilitation and psychiatric distinct part units]
- ☐ ☐ Proposals from the organized medical staff regarding adoption or amendment of medical staff bylaws and/or associated details
- ☐ ☐ Any medical staff bylaws, rules and regulations, and policies that require approval by the governing body
- ☐ ☐ Credentialing process

Medical staff executive committee recommendations
- ☐ ☐ Medical staff membership [CAH, HAP]
- ☐ ☐ Organized medical staff structure [HAP]
- ☐ ☐ Process to review credentials and delineate privileges [HAP]
- ☐ ☐ Delineation of privileges for each practitioner privileged through the medical staff process [CAH only to rehabilitation and psychiatric distinct part units, HAP]
- ☐ ☐ Executive committee review of and actions on reports of medical staff committees, departments, and assigned activity groups [HAP]

Professional graduate medical education committee [HAP]
- ☐ ☐ Safety and quality of patient care, treatment, and services provided by the professional graduate medical education program participants
- ☐ ☐ Related educational and supervisory needs of the professional graduate medical education program participants

Organized medical staff recommendations [CAH, HAP]
- ☐ ☐ Criteria to determine a practitioner's ability to provide patient care, treatment, and services within the scope of the privilege(s) requested
- ☐ ☐ Criteria used to decide to grant, limit, or deny a requested privilege
- ☐ ☐ Clear process for collecting, investigating, and addressing clinical practice concerns

Planning *(board approval, unless noted otherwise)*

✔ N/A
- ☐ ☐ Organization's written scope of services [AHC, BHC, CAH, HAP, LAB, NCC, OME]
- ☐ ☐ Organization's performance in relation to its mission, vision, and goals *(board evaluation required)* [AHC, BHC, CAH, HAP, LAB, NCC, OME]
- ☐ ☐ Organization's mission and vision [CAH, HAP]
- ☐ ☐ Organization's safety and quality goals [CAH, HAP]
- ☐ ☐ Organization's structure and decision-making process [CAH, HAP]
- ☐ ☐ Budget [CAH, HAP]
- ☐ ☐ Population(s) served and related issues *(board discussion required)* [CAH, HAP]
- ☐ ☐ Responsibilities and accountabilities of the governing body, senior managers, and leaders of the organized medical staff, as related to the organization's mission and safety and quality of care [CAH, HAP]
- ☐ ☐ Issues related to safety and quality from senior managers and organized medical staff [CAH, HAP]
- ☐ ☐ Process for managing conflict among leadership groups [CAH, HAP]
- ☐ ☐ Annual operating budget and, when needed, long-term capital expenditure plan [HAP, AHC, BHC, OME]

Accreditation Programs/Settings: AHC = Ambulatory Health Care, BHC = Behavioral Health Care, CAH = Critical Access Hospital, HAP = Hospital, LAB = Laboratory, NCC = Nursing Care Centers, OBS = Office-Based Surgery Practices, OME = Home Care

The E-dition and the comprehensive accreditation manual contain more than just standards. They're full of useful information, including content needed for continuous operational improvement. Important chapters to be aware of include the following:

- ***Patient Safety Systems (PS):*** This chapter, covered in Chapter 2 of this book, gathers quality and safety information from the requirements into one place. It includes descriptions of safety culture, patient safety events, how to become a learning organization, conducting proactive risk assessments, and encouraging patient participation in care, treatment, and services.
- ***The Accreditation Process (ACC):*** This chapter contains details of survey options, scoring, and accreditation decisions.
- ***Sentinel Events (SE):*** This chapter defines sentinel events and explains the Sentinel Event Policy in detail, including how organizations should respond to, report, and follow up on sentinel events and how The Joint Commission reviews and responds to reported sentinel events. The chapter also contains standards related to sentinel events from other parts of the accreditation manual.

The standards and other information are continually under review, and updates are issued twice a year based upon emerging evidence as well as changes from CMS. Each update includes a "What's New" section that lists all the changes since the last update. This makes it easy for organizations to locate relevant changes and respond accordingly. Changes are also announced and noted in *Perspectives*, the official newsletter of The Joint Commission, which publishes monthly and is available to accredited and certified organizations via *Joint Commission Connect* extranet.

CMS Conditions

Organizations that seek Medicare reimbursement must be certified by CMS. To do this, they need to follow the CMS regulations, also known as Conditions of Participation (CoPs) and Conditions for Coverage (CfCs). The State Survey Agency evaluates organizations to determine compliance. Alternately, an organization may use accreditation from a CMS-approved program (such as The Joint Commission) to satisfy the CMS requirements. This is known as "deemed status" (also explained in Chapter 1). Choosing to use accreditation for deemed status purposes allows the organization to undergo one survey for both purposes.

Some Joint Commission standards will vary depending on whether or not the organization is using accreditation for deemed status. These variations are noted throughout E-dition and the *Comprehensive Accreditation Manual.*

Other Government Regulations

Some government organizations have regulatory authority over health care. At the federal level, that includes more than CMS. The Department of Transportation, for example, regulates the transportation of hazardous materials and waste, including those used and generated by health care organizations. The Environmental Protection Agency will also have regulations for handling and disposing of that waste. The Occupational Safety and Health Administration regulates work conditions and worker safety. The US Department of Health and Human Services' Office for Civil Rights oversees the enforcement of the privacy aspects of the Health Insurance Portability and Accountability Act.

Many US federal authorities issue mandates for regulating health care. These include, but aren't limited to, the following:

- Department of Health and Human Services (HHS)
  - Health Resources and Services Administration (HRSA)
  - Office of Inspector General (OIG)
  - Office for Civil Rights (OCR)
  - Office of the National Coordinator for Health Information Technology (ONC)
  - Centers for Medicare & Medicaid Services (CMS)
- Federal Bureau of Investigation (FBI)
- Department of the Treasury (DOT)
  - Internal Revenue Service (IRS)
- Securities and Exchange Commission (SEC)
- Federal Trade Commission (FTC)
- Department of Labor (DOL)
  - Occupational Safety and Health Administration (OSHA)
- Centers for Disease Control and Prevention (CDC)
  - National Institute for Occupational Safety and Health (NIOSH)
- Department of Justice (DOJ)
- Departmental Appeals Board (DAB)
- Environmental Protection Agency (EPA)
- Nuclear Regulatory Commission (NRC)
- Department of Transportation (DOT)
- Federal Aviation Administration (FAA)
- Federal Communications Commission (FCC)
- Department of Consumer Affairs (DCA)
- Food and Drug Administration (FDA)
- Drug Enforcement Administration (DEA)

Organizations must also follow relevant state authorities. These might include licensing agencies, health departments, building and fire codes, workers' rights groups, social service agencies, environmental groups, state attorneys general, and insurance regulators. In addition, local and state governments may adopt regulations created by trade organizations, such as National Fire Protection Association (NFPA), which health care organizations must follow. The Joint Commission and CMS both use NFPA guidelines for life safety (*see* Chapter 1).

Development of a Multidisciplinary Board

As a board member, building awareness of quality and safety regulations—and becoming engaged in patient safety, remaining always accountable, and participating in PI—requires a broad knowledge base. Clinical knowledge is particularly helpful.

Having clinicians as board members is increasingly recognized as an essential component of an effective board. Guidelines from the American Hospital Association recommend that physicians comprise 15%–25% of a hospital board.[18] Similar emphasis is placed on including nursing leaders on boards. Pharmacists are another clinical resource for board membership. But having clinicians on the board is more than just checking a demographic box. Like any board member, clinicians will be effective participants only if their skills are tapped and their perspectives valued.[19]

Call to Action
Development of a Multidisciplinary Board

Diversity is critical to an effective board. Physicians and nurses offer knowledge diversity, but other types of diversity are equally important. Individuals of varying age, ethnicity, culture, and sexual orientation offer unique perspectives on issues and create a robust base for discussion. As a board member, seek out and welcome new members with different backgrounds than yours. At the very least, look at the populations your organization serves and strive for representation of those groups among board members.

Seeking Physician Leadership and Insight

Much is said about taking a multidisciplinary approach to assembling committees for PI, risk assessments, and other safety issues. Diversity of experience, knowledge, and focus is invaluable when addressing complex problems and situations. Engaging a variety of people in any process minimizes the risk of something being overlooked or misinterpreted.

The same applies to a board of directors. Leadership, governance, and business training are all important skills to have. But, as reimbursement is increasingly linked to quality-of-care metrics, boards need clinical perspectives on safety to inform new business strategies. Physicians, as well as other clinicians, can provide these valuable insights.[19]

Clinicians can also offer unique perspectives on quality improvement efforts, patient experiences, and other issues that affect safety. For example, physicians interact with patients and staff members every day. They have practical knowledge and firsthand experiences that other board members may lack.[19]

The Case Study on page 134 shows how one organization has developed a unique way of involving physicians and other clinical leaders on its board.

Valuing Nurse Experience and Adaptability

Despite their critical role in patient care, nurses make up only about 2% of hospital board members.[20] Many organizations feel this needs to change. For example, the former Institute of Medicine (the National Academies of Medicine) states that nurses must be active in boards and other policy-making positions in order to improve patient care.[21] Several reasons are cited for why a nurse is a valuable addition to a board, including the following:

- ***Patient contact and communications:*** First, nurses often spend the most time physically delivering care to and interacting with patients. This puts nurses in the unique position to know the patients' needs and how they are (or are not) being met.[22] Nurses' frequent interactions with patients also gives them valuable communication skills. Nurses are used to explaining complex clinical concepts to patients; this skill can be applicable in board discussions, too, particularly with other members who come from nonmedical backgrounds.[22]

continued on page 136

• CASE STUDY •

Clinicians as Board Members

WHO THEY ARE

Aurora Health Care is a system of 15 hospitals, more than 150 clinics, and 70 pharmacies. Headquartered n Milwaukee, Wisconsin, it serves 30 communities throughout eastern Wisconsin and northern Illinois.

WHAT THEY DID

The system downsized and reorganized its board in 2007. Previously, the board consisted of 21 members from both inside and outside the organization. Now, the board has 11 members, all of whom fly in from other, out-of-state organizations. The only internal physician board member is the system president and CEO, who is an ex officio member.

These changes didn't mean that Aurora Health Care reduced its input from physicians. The system still maintains two positions on its board specifically for clinical experts: one for a physician and one for a nurse. And the board's quality and safety committee is led by the physician member. In addition to these voting positions, the board seeks clinical expertise from physicians and nursing leaders through their committee system. Physicians and nurses alike are heavily involved in the board's committees, not just regarding quality but also the finance, social responsibility, and other committees. These participants, who are drawn from across the Aurora Health Care system, provide input and engage board members in dialogue on every issue the board addresses.

A leadership development program. Aurora Health Care has also instituted a leadership development program for physicians, nurses, and administrative staff who are seen as emerging leaders within the system. These individuals participate in a structured curriculum that centers on hands-on quality improvement activities. Each participant designs and conducts an "action project" under the guidance of a mentor and with a strong support structure. For a year or more, they identify performance gaps, design interventions, measure results, and track progress. Since the program's inception in 2011, more than 120 people have completed the curriculum.

THEIR RESULTS

Aurora Health Care has long recognized the importance of clinical input on a board. This was a particular concern during the system's downsizing and restructuring. The system did not want to lose clinical input, which would compromise its quality and safety goals, particularly when developing long-term strategies as a health care system.

Aurora Health Care has seen numerous advantages to its purposeful involvement of physicians and nurses in the board and its activities. For one, clinical input is brought to the forefront. Also, the board's discussions about quality and patient safety are richer. Physicians "bring the patient voice into the boardroom," helping the board members without a clinical background to better understand the realities of providing care.

It works in reverse as well. Incorporating physician representatives into all committees has the benefit of giving physicians a perspective on investments, property, strategic partnerships, and other nonclinical issues. This perspective gives them insight into the board's decisions—insight they can take back to their colleagues.

Respecting perspectives. Gaining this perspective can be a challenge for all board members. Everyone brings his or her own expertise and background to the discussion, which provides needed diversity. However, it's important for members to make a conscious attempt to understand and respect the perspectives of their fellow members—and it's an opportunity for board members to learn from each other and grow together.

This can be an uncomfortable process, particularly for physicians, as it may be their first experience with sitting on a board. But that's a driving force behind the leadership development program: It exposes the participants to these issues so they aren't new. This way, they can be ready to engage on their first day.

A powerful way to learn. The leadership development program's hands-on component also has benefits for the quality and patient safety at Aurora Health Care facilities. Not only do these action projects directly improve care, they give participants a firsthand perspective on what safety is and how it can be improved. Participants in the program are applying knowledge to actual work and making actual improvements in the health system—and they've found that's a powerful way to learn.

- ***Frontline implementation across the care continuum:*** Nurses also have a unique view of how care is provided. Their roles take them into various settings across the continuum of care, which provides a systemwide perspective that is extremely valuable to organizational leadership.[23] Also, as the clinicians on the front lines of care, nurses are generally the ones who put the board's policy changes into action. When nurses are involved in designing those changes, they can improve buy-in from nursing staff—which leads to sustainable change.[22]
- ***Adaptability in the shifting industry:*** Finally, nurses will be key players as the health care industry continues to change. As health care shifts to a value-based care system, nurses can help identify opportunities to reduce waste and improve the patient experience.[22] In addition, their education in wellness and health promotion will grow in importance as the health care industry continues to shift in that direction.[23]

Bias and gender obstacles. In short, nurses can add a diversity of knowledge, experience, and perspective to a board that is crucial to effective governing. Despite these benefits, nurses' skill and expertise are often dismissed as irrelevant to board operations, or undervalued by organizations and even the nurses themselves.[23] Gender may also play a role. Board membership at nonprofit and public hospitals, for example, is estimated to be only 23% women, while an estimated 90% of nurses in the United States are women.[20] Overcoming these obstacles can result in boards significantly benefiting from trustees who are nurses.

Recognizing Pharmacist Expertise and Management

As discussed in Chapter 1, pharmacists are becoming more active in patient care as they manage complex medication therapies. Further, pharmacist leaders have the clinical expertise and management skills that are increasingly recognized as useful to board discussions and decisions. And yet, pharmacists are often overlooked as board members. Organizations should consider ways of encouraging pharmacist leaders to pursue leadership training opportunities to help them prepare for effective board membership.[24]

Development of an Effective Board

Simply recruiting clinical leaders, including physicians and nurses, to the board doesn't make them effective board members, of course. The individual may have served successfully in leadership roles within the organization, in medical associations, and other groups, yet struggle to transition to the unique culture of an organization board. What makes a clinician a good departmental leader may work against him or her in the boardroom. The dynamics, hierarchy, culture, and expectations of a board can be confusing or intimidating for clinicians, even when the board makes an effort to provide orientation.[25]

Governing vs. Managing

One reason clinicians may be ineffective board members lies in the distinction between governing and managing. For example, physicians are used to managing their practice: assessing a situation (diagnosing an illness) and giving directions on how to address it (for example, prescribing treatments and diagnostics). This is appropriate when providing care, but it doesn't translate well into the board environment.[25] And nurse leaders often supervise large numbers of people and manage a significant budget.[23] They're frequently expected to make rapid, critical decisions on patient care resources and interprofessional situations.

Instead of giving directions, board members provide direction. They work with large-scale concepts like "mission" and "vision" to provide governance. This can be difficult for physicians, nurses, and other clinical leaders, who are used to the more concrete and tangible act of managing. They must shift to a collaborative, persuasive, communicative approach among equals.[25]

Not just subject matter experts. Treating clinicians as board members, not just representatives of their profession, is important to remember.[23] It can be a challenge for clinicians to focus on governing and avoid managing, particularly when an issue addresses their area of expertise. Similarly, nonclinician members may view clinicians as subject matter resources rather than full board members. In sum, board members who come from clinical backgrounds should function as board members who are clinicians, and not as clinicians who are board members. It's a fine line, but a crucial one.

Admitting Limitations

Clinicians often come to board membership with a reluctance to admit their own limitations or ignorance. This is understandable—no patient wants to hear his or her doctor or nurse say "I don't know." But boards must deal with issues, like finances and regulatory mandates, something clinicians without management background may have little to no experience dealing with. Clinicians may also lack the leadership and business education and experience that other board members have. It can be a challenge to admit these limitations, especially to new colleagues.[19]

Of course, no one can know everything about everything. All board members must view board participation as a collaborative learning experience. Doing this taps into clinicians' natural talent and desire for learning—the exact talent and desire that helped them become clinical leaders in the first place. Board leadership should ensure that the board's culture is one in which members recognize their own strengths and limitations, are receptive to others' perspectives, and are comfortable speaking up when their area of expertise is applicable.[19]

Trusting and Communicating

Trust is an essential component for any effective board, particularly as it applies to involving clinicians. This trust must flow in several directions. Clinician board members must trust others to be able to admit their limitations, and nonclinician board members must trust that the physicians, nurses, and pharmacists are bringing valuable experience to the group.[25]

Trust is based on communication. Misunderstanding between clinician and nonclinician board members may occur over their respective knowledge bases. Nonclinicians will assume clinicians know more (or less) than they do, and vice versa. This is avoided when board members engage in open communication. Transparency also eliminates political and personal motivations, which are detrimental to good decision making and undermine trust.[25]

Development of a Learning Board

Learning to feel comfortable in new roles of responsibility—and learning new content areas to make better decisions—is a part of the changing health care scene. Health care is a complex and dynamic system with many moving parts that interact and change frequently. If organizations are going to provide high-quality care, they must adapt to reflect those changes. Boards must guide their organizations in new directions. To do this, they must stay ahead of the curve and continually educate themselves on the latest and upcoming health care issues, regulatory mandates, and governance practices.

Given the complexity of health care, no one board member will know everything there is to know about every issue that will be on the agenda. Each person will have different strengths and weaknesses depending on his or her background. This is a good thing, because complex issues require diverse perspectives to lead to good decisions. But it also means that everyone has room to learn, and a diverse board offers the perfect opportunity to do so. Recognizing and admitting one's knowledge gaps is vitally important. Yet again, it's only truly possible in a culture of safety, trust, and transparency.

To read about how one hospital has developed a board education program dedicated to patient safety and high reliability principles, *see* the Case Study on page 140.

Bringing in a Quality and Safety Expert

Because quality and safety is a relatively recent requirement for a governing body's responsibilities, many board members don't have specific training or experience with those issues. It can be helpful to enlist a quality and safety expert to guide and educate the board.

Chief quality officer. Organizations are increasingly relying on a chief quality officer. This individual will have high-level responsibility for a number of tasks related to quality and safety improvement. Depending on the needs of the particular organization, these tasks might include the following[26]:

- Collecting and reporting data
- Identifying and implementing improvement initiatives
- Fostering a culture in which quality is prioritized throughout the organization
- Collaborating with other leaders on quality issues
- Strengthening data collection systems and analysis methods

This individual will be a valuable resource for boards looking to better understand quality data, improvement initiatives, and so on.

Listening to Frontline Staff

Another valuable resource for boards is the organization's frontline staff. These individuals deal with the day-to-day implementation of the policies and initiatives that originate with the board. They also have intimate knowledge of how the processes and procedures work, and often recognize weaknesses that might not show up in data analysis.

One way to seek information from frontline staff is to invite them to speak at board meetings. This may be part of the board's routine quality discussion, or in response to a particular issue on which the board needs guidance. Doing this

continued on page 142

• CASE STUDY •

Educating the Board on Safety

WHO THEY ARE

Memorial Hermann Health System in Texas has 13 hospitals and numerous specialty programs in the greater Houston area. This not-for-profit organization, the largest in southeast Texas, has 5,500 affiliated physicians and 24,000 employees.

WHAT THEY DID

About 10 years ago, Memorial Hermann made a conscious decision to make safety a priority. The organization started by assessing its core values. This resulted in safety being declared the system's only core value. The organization's leaders knew that this wasn't enough to affect real, sustainable improvements. At the time, the board was comprised of primarily lay community leaders with backgrounds in business, investments, and property management. Their knowledge of providing care and the importance of safety was limited. Memorial Hermann recognized that this needed to change. A section on quality and safety was incorporated into the orientation course that all board members completed. In addition, all board members attended a yearly educational forum presented by the Institute for Healthcare Improvement (IHI) called "From the Top: The Role of the Board in Quality and Safety."

Memorial Hermann had much success with this program, and when it was discontinued in late 2014, they created their own version. Now the system brings in quality and safety experts to run a daylong program for board members, board committee members, physician leaders, and others. The only topic of this session is quality and safety.

Focusing on high reliability. The central component of Memorial Hermann's focus on safety is the adoption of high reliability principles (*see* Chapter 2 for more information on high reliability). Part of this effort was the identification of two simple goals that apply to every facility it operates. The first goal is 100% compliance with quality guidelines, and the second is a 0% incidence of adverse events, such as health care–associated infections (HAIs). Achieving these goals was incorporated into the system's incentive program.

Supporting the high reliability goals was the creation of an active System Quality Committee. All safety improvement–related activities from every corner of the system are accountable to this overarching committee. The

System Quality Committee is chaired by a physician member of the board. This individual provides a complete safety report at every board meeting. Any safety issues unresolved at the committee level are presented to the whole board for discussion.

THEIR RESULTS

Since adopting the concept of high reliability and initiating its processes, Memorial Hermann has seen significant safety improvements. For example, the system targeted HAIs, in part, by partnering with the Joint Commission Center for Transforming Healthcare in its efforts to promote reliable hand hygiene behaviors. This resulted in the system's average hand hygiene compliance rate improving from 44% in 2007 to 92% in 2013.

Zero adverse events. By 2011 Memorial Hermann had hospitals reporting 0% yearly incidence rates for a number of specific adverse events. In response, the system created the "Certified Zero Award" for hospitals that have zero occurrences of the various adverse events (central line infections, for example). Memorial Hermann has awarded 186 Certified Zero Awards to various system hospitals for specific adverse events.

The organization has realized that changing the focus of the board to quality and safety is difficult, but necessary, noting that it doesn't work as a grassroots effort, but has to come from the top down, which means engaging the board.

High reliability helps everything fall into place. Memorial Hermann's success with implementing high reliability principles is made possible through its board education program. The focus on safety is primary in everything the board does. The organization's theory is that if they achieve high reliability, everything else will fall in place: finances, patient satisfaction, employee engagement, and so on.

Memorial Hermann has consciously designed its safety education program to be more relatable to board members. One way the system has done this is by utilizing board members who are already enthusiastic and passionate about safety. These individuals are invited to be presenters or instructors at orientation or education forums. It's just one more way they've found success in engaging as well as educating their board.

encourages trust and accountability in the organization, underscoring the board's prioritization of quality.

Another way to learn from frontline staff is to attend clinical team meetings. At some organizations, board members request permission to attend meetings of physicians, nutritionists, radiologists, and other specialists. This can give board members greater knowledge of not only the individual departments but also how they all work together.[27] This can lead to better perspectives on systemwide safety and quality as well as issues such as efficiency, patient flow, workflow, and others.

Soliciting Patient Testimonials

Another potential source of information are the patients themselves. Boards may want to ask the administration to include patients and their family members in the quality and safety section of your agenda. Patient opinions can be solicited through satisfaction surveys, presented through video or in-person testimonials, or shared by board members or administrators who have worked directly with patients.

Patients and family members have a unique perspective on how an organization delivers care. Their experiences can be extremely powerful, because they put a "human face" on abstract concepts, demonstrating real-world consequences in a way that performance data review cannot.

Call to Action
Soliciting Patient Testimonials

There's a difference between data and information. Data are raw numbers; information is the application of critical analysis to make sense of those numbers. Seeking personal experiences of patients and staff can help boards make sense of performance data. These stories can create in trustees a personal connection to the issue at hand. When that happens, the trustees become invested in the issue, and finding a solution gains importance. The satisfaction of helping real people translates to motivation to continue doing just that.

Finding Additional Learning Opportunities

Learning should not be limited to "special occasions" like an annual conference. Boards must strive to continually develop their knowledge, understanding, and perspectives.[27] Educational development can take many forms. Leaders can provide the board with relevant written materials, such as reports, studies, and articles. Video presentations or Web-based programs can be incorporated into board meetings. Board members can attend conferences, retreats, lectures, and other organizations' meetings to gain additional perspective. The type of activity is less important than the engagement of the board members in ongoing education opportunities.[27] (This book itself also would serve as a useful orientation guide for new board members and/or a refresher for existing board members.)

Even boards that are already familiar with quality and safety will benefit from continuing education. Regulations, standards of care, and clinical or technological innovations are constantly changing. Continuing education on these and other topics can suggest new areas for consideration or raise the level of expectations for improvement.

The Next Step

Patience, commitment, enthusiasm, motivation, and the willingness to learn—these are some of the qualities board members need as they push organizations toward safer, higher-quality care. There will be challenges, but this is a normal part of the journey toward the ultimate goal of providing the safest and the highest-quality care possible.

Board members have many opportunities to lead by example. The interest that health care board members like yourself show in quality and safety issues will be mirrored in the efforts of senior leaders and staff to improve processes and systems. Whether trustees are demanding higher goals for quality and safety initiatives, encouraging transparency in reporting, or celebrating the successes of improvement teams, they're showing both internal and external stakeholders that quality and safety are top priorities in the organization.

REFERENCES

1. Tsai TC, et al. Hospital board and management practices are strongly related to hospital performance on clinical quality metrics. Health Aff (Millwood). 2015 Aug;34(8):1304–1311.
2. HealthLeaders Media. Active Hospital Boards Linked to Better Clinical Outcomes. Boivin J. Aug 10, 2015. Accessed Aug 28, 2016. http://healthleadersmedia.com/page-1/QUA-319419/Active-Hospital-Boards-Linked-to-Better-Clinical-Outcomes##.
3. National Patient Safety Foundation (NPSF), Lucian Leape Institute. Shining a Light: Safer Health Care Through Transparency. Boston: NPSF, 2015.
4. Walker L. Governance never events. Trustee. 2013 Jan;66(1):6–7.
5. Combes JR, Totten MK, Prybil LD. Helping boards achieve and demonstrate accountability: Taking responsibility to new levels. Healthc Exec. 2014 May–Jun;29(3):76, 78.
6. Evans M. Bonuses still tied to better financials. Use of CEO pay incentives for quality is uneven across for-profit hospital systems. Mod Healthc. 2014 Apr 28;44(17):12–15. Accessed Aug 28, 2016. http://www.modernhealthcare.com/article/20140426/MAGAZINE/304269985.
7. Sandler M. Going up: Surge in exec comp driven by pay-for-performance bonuses. Mod Healthc. 2015 Aug 10;45(32):18–22. Accessed Aug 28, 2016. http://www.modernhealthcare.com/article/20150808/MAGAZINE/308089987.
8. Health Affairs. Health Policy Briefs: Pay-for-Performance. Oct 11, 2012. Accessed Aug 28, 2016. http://www.healthaffairs.org/healthpolicybriefs/brief.php?brief_id=78.
9. The Physicians Foundation. 2014 Survey of America's Physicians: Practice Patterns & Perspectives. Sep 2014. Accessed Aug 28, 2016. http://www.physiciansfoundation.org/uploads/default/2014_Physicians_Foundation_Biennial_Physician_Survey_Report.pdf.
10. Becker's Hospital Review. Shifting Cultures: A Change Management Guide for Hospital Leaders. Herman B. Nov 22, 2011. Accessed Aug 28, 2016. http://www.beckershospitalreview.com/hospital-management-administration/shifting-cultures-a-change-management-guide-for-hospital-leaders.html.
11. Büchner VA, Schreyögg J, Schultz C. The impact of the board's strategy-setting role on board-management relations and hospital performance. Health Care Manage Rev. 2014 Oct–Dec;39(4):305–317.
12. Hinna A, Scarozza D. A behavioral perspective for governing bodies: Processes and conflicts in public organizations. International Studies of Management & Organization. 2015;45(1):43–59.
13. Schyve PM. Leadership in Healthcare Organizations: A Guide to Joint Commission Leadership Standards. A Governance Institute white paper. San Diego: The Governance Institute, 2009. Accessed Aug 28, 2016. http://www.jointcommission.org/assets/1/18/wp_leadership_standards.pdf.
14. US Department of Health and Human Services, Office of Inspector General. Practical Guidance for Health Care Governing Boards on Compliance Oversight. Matos K, et al. Apr 20, 2015. Accessed Aug 28, 2016. https://oig.hhs.gov/compliance/compliance-guidance/docs/Practical-Guidance-for-Health-Care-Boards-on-Compliance-Oversight.pdf.
15. Pugh M, Reinertsen J. Reducing harm to patients: Using patient safety dashboards at the board level. Healthc Exec. 2007 Nov–Dec;22(6):62, 64–65.
16. Huff C. Board dashboards deliver vital stats: Evolving board dashboards capture key metrics. Trustee. 2015 Sep;68(8):8–12.
17. Goeschel CA, et al. Board quality scorecards: Measuring improvement. Am J Med Qual. 2011 Jul–Aug;26(4):254–260.

18. Scott BC. Hospital boards: Why quality and safety matter. Physician Leadersh J. 2015 Jan–Feb;2(1):62–64.

19. Physician leadership and governance. Trustee. 2014 Sep;67(8):45–47.

20. Rose T, Nies MA. A place at the table: Positioning nurses where healthcare decisions are made. Nurs Manage. 2016 Jan;47(1):42–46.

21. Institute of Medicine. The Future of Nursing: Leading Change, Advancing Health. Washington, DC: National Academies Press, 2011.

22. Becker's Hospital Review. 5 Reasons Hospital Boards Need More Nurses. Barnet S. Dec 8, 2014. Accessed Aug 28, 2016. http://www.beckershospitalreview.com/hospital-management-administration/5-reasons-hospital-boards-need-more-nurses.html.

23. Brown L. Educating nurse leaders for board service: The Northwest Organization of Nurse Executives' story. Nurs Adm Q. 2015 Jan–Mar;39(1):28–31.

24. American Hospital Association (AHA), Center for Healthcare Governance. 2014 National Health Care Governance Survey Report. Chicago: AHA Center for Healthcare Governance, 2014. Accessed Aug 28, 2016. http://www.americangovernance.com/resources/reports/governance-reports/2014/Governance-Survey-Report-update.pdf.

25. Hernandez J. Serving on boards: Caveats for physician leaders. Physician Leadersh J. 2014 Sep–Oct;1(1):72–76.

26. Becker's Hospital Review. What Makes an 'Ideal' Chief Quality Officer? Barnet S. Jun 30, 2015. Accessed Dec 28, 2016. http://www.beckershospitalreview.com/quality/what-makes-an-ideal-chief-quality-officer.html.

27. Bush H. Creating a culture of safety. Trustee. 2013 Jul–Aug;66(7):8–12. Accessed Aug 28, 2016. http://www.trusteemag.com/articles/91-creating-a-culture-of-safety.

Glossary

accreditation Determination by The Joint Commission that an eligible organization complies with applicable Joint Commission accreditation requirements.

accreditation manual A Joint Commission publication consisting of policies, procedures, and accreditation requirements relating to ambulatory care, behavioral health care, critical access hospital, home care, hospital, nursing care centers, office-based surgery centers, and clinical laboratory and point-of-care testing. Organizations should use the manual that contains the set of accreditation requirements most appropriate to their primary focus or mission of the organization.

accreditation process A continuous process whereby organizations are required to demonstrate to The Joint Commission that they are providing safe, high-quality care, as determined by compliance with Joint Commission standards, National Patient Safety Goals, and performance measurement requirements (as applicable). Key components of this process are an on-site evaluation of the organization by a Joint Commission surveyor(s) and, where applicable, quarterly submission of performance measurement data to The Joint Commission.

adverse drug event (ADE) An injury resulting from a medical intervention related to a medication, including harm from an adverse drug reaction or a medication error.

adverse event A patient safety event that resulted in harm to a patient.

behaviors that undermine a culture of safety Conduct by staff working in the organization that intimidates others to the extent that quality and safety could be compromised. These behaviors, as determined by the organization, may be verbal or nonverbal, may involve the use of rude language, may be threatening, or may involve physical contact.

board The individual(s), group, or agency that has ultimate authority and responsibility for establishing policy; maintaining quality of care, treatment, or services; and providing for organization management and planning. Other names for this group include governance, board of trustees, board of governors, board of commissioners, and governing body.

clinical leader An individual with essential clinical knowledge who sets expectations, develops plans, and implements procedures to assess and improve the quality of the organization's clinical and support functions and processes.

clinical staff Individuals such as employees, licensed independent practitioners, contractors, volunteers, or temporary agency personnel who provide or have provided clinical services to the organization's patients, residents, or individual served.

close call A patient safety event that did not reach the patient; also called near miss or good catch.

comprehensive systematic analysis A process for identifying basic or causal factors underlying variation in performance, including the occurrence or possible occurrence of a sentinel event. A root cause analysis is one type of comprehensive systematic analysis.

culture of safety An environment in which safety is the top priority. In a culture of safety, not only are processes designed for optimal safety but also employees feel safe in reporting unsafe situations. Also referred to as a *safety culture.*

deemed status Status conferred by the Centers for Medicare & Medicaid Services (CMS) on an organization whose standards and survey process are determined by CMS to be equivalent to those of the Medicare program or other federal laws, such as the Clinical Laboratory Improvement Amendments of 1988 (CLIA

'88). Accreditation is voluntary and seeking deemed status through accreditation is an option, not a requirement.

E-dition® A web-based electronic version of current Joint Commission accreditation standards, including all related content printed in the *Comprehensive Accreditation Manual.*

element of performance (EP) Specific action(s), process(es), or structure(s) that must be implemented to achieve the goal of a standard. The scoring of EP compliance determines an organization's overall compliance with a standard.

Emergency Operations Plan (EOP) An organization's written document that describes the process it would implement for managing the consequences of emergencies, including natural and human-made disasters, that could disrupt the organization's ability to provide care, treatment, and services.

Evidence of Standards Compliance (ESC) A report that a surveyed organization must submit after a survey in which it receives a Requirement for Improvement (RFI) for an accreditation requirement. The report must detail actions taken to bring the organization into compliance with the requirement, or explain why the organization believes it's in compliance. A corrective ESC must address compliance at the EP level for all applicable corrections and be submitted within 60 days after a survey. If the organization believes it was in compliance at the time of survey, it may submit a clarifying ESC, which includes an explanation and proof of compliance. The clarifying ESC must be submitted within 10 business days following the posting of the organization's report on the extranet.

Focused Standards Assessment (FSA) A required standards self-assessment designed to help organizations maintain continuous compliance.

hazard vulnerability analysis (HVA) A process for identifying potential emergencies and how they may affect the health care organization's ability to care for patients, given its size, geographic location, proximity to sources of danger, and so on.

health care–associated infection (HAI) An infection acquired concomitantly by an individual who is receiving or has received care, treatment, or services from a health care organization. The infection may or may not have resulted from the care, treatment, or services.

high reliability An indication of a low level of poor outcomes despite a high level of hazardous conditions, achieved through use of leadership commitment to zero patient harm, a fully functional safety culture, and Robust Process Improvement® (RPI®) methods.

high-risk procedures or processes A procedure or process that, if not planned and/or implemented correctly, has a significant potential for affecting the safety of a patient or an individual served.

interim life safety measures (ILSM) A set of administrative actions intended to temporarily compensate for significant hazards posed by existing National Fire Protection Association *Life Safety Code*®* deficiencies or construction activities.

Intracycle Monitoring (ICM) A process that helps accredited organizations maintain continuous compliance through a self-assessment of high-risk areas and related standards. It involves use of the organization's ICM Profile available on the organization's *Joint Commission Connect*™ extranet site.

leader An individual who sets expectations, develops plans, and implements procedures to assess and improve the quality of the organization's governance, management, and clinical and support functions and processes. At a minimum, leaders include members of the governing body and medical staff, the chief executive officer and other senior managers, the nurse executive, clinical leaders, and staff members in leadership positions within the organization.

leadership group Individuals in senior positions with clearly defined, unique responsibilities. These might include governance, management, medical staff, and clinical staff. Not every organization will have all these groups, and an individual may be a member of more than one group.

* *Life Safety Code*® is a registered trademark of the National Fire Protection Association, Quincy, MA.

Life Safety Code® A set of standards for the construction and operation of buildings intended to provide a reasonable degree of safety during fires. These standards are prepared, published, and periodically revised by the National Fire Protection Association and adopted by The Joint Commission to evaluate health care organizations under its life safety management program.

medical staff The group of all licensed independent practitioners and other practitioners privileged through the organized medical staff process that is subject to the medical staff bylaws. This group may include others, such as retired practitioners who no longer practice in the organization but who wish to continue their membership in the group, courtesy staff, scientific staff, and so forth.

medication error A preventable event that may cause or lead to inappropriate medication use or patient or resident harm while the medication is in the control of the health care professional, patient, resident, or consumer. Such events may be related to professional practice, health care products, procedures, and systems, including prescribing; order communication; product labeling, packaging, and nomenclature; compounding; dispensing; distribution; administration; education; monitoring; and use.

multidisciplinary team A group of staff members composed of representatives from a range of professions, disciplines, or service areas

nurse executive A registered professional nurse who is responsible for the full-time, direct supervision of nursing services and who is currently licensed by the state in which he or she practices. Attributes of this position may be further defined in regulatory statues.

outcome measure A tool used to assess data that indicates the results of performance or nonperformance of a function or procedure

patient safety event An event, incident, or condition that could have or did result in harm to a patient.

performance improvement The systematic process of detecting and analyzing performance problems, designing and developing interventions to address the problems, implementing the interventions, evaluating the results, and sustaining improvement.

performance measurement A method of gauging organization performance that facilitates improvement through the collection of data and information and the dissemination of process and/or outcome measures over time.

process measure A measure that focuses on one or more steps that lead to a certain outcome.

quality of care, treatment, and services The degree to which care, treatment, or services for individuals and populations increases the likelihood of desired health or behavioral health outcomes. Considerations include the appropriateness, efficacy, efficiency, timeliness, accessibility, and continuity of care; the safety of the care environment; and the individual's personal values, practices, and beliefs.

Requirement for Improvement (RFI) A recommendation that an organization must address in its Evidence of Standards Compliance (ESC) report in order to retain accreditation.

risk assessment, proactive An assessment that examines a process in detail including sequencing of events, actual and potential risks, and failure or points of vulnerability and that prioritizes, through a logical process, areas for improvement based on the actual or potential impact (that is, criticality) of care, treatment, or services provided.

safety The degree to which the risk of an intervention (for example, use of a drug, or a procedure) and risk in the care environment are reduced for a patient and other persons, including health care practitioners. Safety risks may arise from the performance of tasks, from the structure of the physical environment, or from situations beyond the organization's control (such as weather).

safety management Activities selected and implemented by the organization to assess and control the impact of environmental risk, and to improve general environmental safety.

sentinel event A patient safety event (not primarily related to the natural course of the patient's illness or underlying condition) that reaches a patient and results in death, permanent harm, or severe temporary harm. Sentinel events are a subcategory of adverse events.

standard A principle of patient safety and quality of care that a well-run organization meets. A standard defines the performance expectations, structures, or processes that must be substantially in place in an organization to enhance the quality of care, treatment, or services.

The Joint Commission An independent, not-for-profit organization dedicated to improving the safety and quality of health care through standards development, public policy initiatives, accreditation, and certification. The Joint Commission accredits and certifies more than 20,000 health care organizations and programs in the United States.

tracer methodology A process surveyors use during the on-site survey to analyze an organization's systems or processes for delivering safe, high-quality care by following an individual patient or resident through the organization's care process in the sequence experienced by each individual. Depending on the setting, this process may require surveyors to visit multiple care programs and services within an organization or within a single program or service to "trace" the care rendered.

Index

B

C

D

E

F

H

M

N

O

U

W

Z